Jenny Phillips has a first D̶e̶... ̶B̶A from Henley Business Schoo̶l̶ ... ̶dicine. She is also a qualifie̶...

Originally from a ma̶... ̶c̶kground, she undertook a career cha̶... ̶a̶s after seeing first-hand the success of an i̶n̶... ̶o̶ach to recover from her own experience with cance̶r̶...

Since qualifying in 2010 Jenny has worked extensively with clients to help them to recover optimal health. She has great success at motivating and enabling people to make sustainable lifestyle changes. She has a wide breadth of experience, providing nutritional advice that complements mainstream treatments.

In light of her own personal experience, Jenny resonates with people going through cancer at any stage of their journey. In addition to private appointments, she works with two charities – Together Against Cancer and Yes to Life – to deliver *Outsmart Cancer* workshops and cookery classes.

Jenny is a health writer and public speaker, and regularly blogs at www.InspiredNutrition.co.uk. Here you can follow her on social media, sign up for news updates and contact her to make private appointments. She also runs retreats, where you can enjoy a short time of health indulgence, in both the UK and Europe.

"I was convinced my autoimmune condition and subsequent inflammation must have played a role in how my cancer developed. Fortunately, Jenny was there as an alternative adjunct to what I was getting from my conventional doctors and was able to provide me with a nutrition program that complimented my main-stream therapy. She is experienced at dealing with cancer, well versed in the theories and ideas for treating it and was able to provide many useful leads for high quality supplements. Jenny is firmly in the "common sense" camp, practicing safe, conservative alternate medicine."
Greg Allwood, 2015

Eat to

OUTSMART

Cancer

How to create optimal health
for prevention & recovery

JENNY PHILLIPS

Eat to *Outsmart Cancer*

First published in Great Britain in 2015 by Completely Novel

ISBN 9781849147170

Text design and typeset by Emma Hiwaizi

Diagrams by Joanna Rucklidge

Back cover photo by www.JoScottImages.co.uk

www.completelynovel.com

Disclaimer

This book is for educational purposes only and is not to be taken as medical advice or instruction. You should consult your own physician or a qualified health professional on any matters regarding your health or on any opinions expressed within this book. The information provided is believed to be accurate based on the best knowledge of the author, who assumes no responsibility for unwitting errors, omissions or inaccuracies. The author will not accept any responsibility for the actions or consequential results of any action taken by you, the reader. If you have active cancer, always consult your oncology team before embarking on a supplement regime.

Acknowledgements

Deciding to write a book is one thing, but actually seeing it through the ups and downs is quite another. I am extremely appreciative of the support of Karen Williams, who excels in coaching people through this challenging yet rewarding process. Karen - your expert eye, knowledge of publishing and motivation are priceless.

The one person who has been with me right through this project is Emma Hiwaizi. She took on board the copy editing and design, and has also been an integral part of the development of the content. Her critical eye, courage to challenge and great ideas have made a significant impact on the final edition and it has been a pleasure to work with her. We met on a raw food retreat in France two years ago, where neither of us could have foreseen that we would be working together in this way.

Thank you too for the feedback given freely by many of my friends and colleagues, in particular Dr Xandria Williams, Dr Tanya Malpass, Amanda Gillies, Angela May, Sarah Paton and Marta Krumina.

Melanie and Steve Gamble have helped to bring this book to life by supporting OUTSMART Cancer workshops. These have been generously funded by the charity Together Against Cancer, which has enabled cancer patients to attend free of charge.

Finally, I am eternally grateful for the opportunity to work with so many enlightened people, who are striving to make significant health improvements and are sometimes in difficult places. We should all learn from them, and live each day as the gift that it was intended to be.

Contents

Foreword

By Robin Daly, founder and chairman of cancer charity, Yes to Life

Something is going fundamentally wrong with the health of our nation. Chronic, debilitating disease, and particularly cancer, is on an unprecedented runaway trajectory. I personally am in no doubt that the underlying causes are the very recent changes in the way we live: what we eat and drink, our day to day activities, our habitual stress levels, our home, work and other environments.

Of the many lifestyle factors that can contribute to our health, or lack of it, nutrition has the potential to serve us a 'double whammy' if we get it wrong. Poor choices in nutrition, typically highly processed and denatured foods, contain a plethora of added chemicals, all deemed 'safe' for human consumption by the authorities, but many of which are known to be toxic or carcinogenic, cancer promoting. These same foods are likely to have the lowest nutritional content, depriving us of the very fuel we require to combat these toxins.

Jenny Phillips is a powerhouse of enthusiasm and knowledge about good nutrition. She is passionate about the insights that she feels have provided her with the basis for another way of living, and she urgently wants to communicate this knowledge to empower as many others as possible. Her prompt to learn and to make these changes herself was cancer, and she determined to give herself the very best chance of a long and healthy life by extending the standard of care she received from the NHS, and including a re-evaluation of every aspect of her life that had led her to be so unwell in the first place.

This approach, which, besides nutrition, can include exercise, complementary therapies, psycho-social support and more, is now termed integrative medicine, or, more specifically with cancer, integrative oncology. By extending care beyond normal orthodox approaches such as surgery or chemotherapy, the attention pans out from a narrow focus on a tumour or symptoms, to encompass the whole person, and their lifestyle choices. This change has the effect of putting a 'victim of cancer' right back in the driving seat of their lives, making positive choices for good health - a radically different stance that can have far reaching consequences for their future. At Yes to Life, our belief is that integrative oncology is the future of cancer medicine, and so we are supporting people in accessing its benefits, following in the footsteps of some other progressive countries.

Possibly the most valuable pearl contained within the message of integrative oncology is the direct link between the way we live and long term health. This message has the power to turn the tide of chronic conditions and to become a potent public health message, that prevention is a genuine possibility - if we are equipped with the right information. When it comes to nutrition, that information is right here in *Eat to Outsmart Cancer*, giving us the potential to outsmart cancer before we even get it, as well as if we have it, or if we are determined to prevent a recurrence.

Jenny's passion and excitement for good nutrition leap off the page, and her writing style is engaging and accessible, making *Eat to Outsmart Cancer* an easy and compelling read. The down to earth, practical advice and information it contains will satisfy anyone who is hungry for ways to improve their odds against cancer.

Introduction

When I was at Management College in my early thirties, we gave a presentation on a subject of our choice. For some reason, I chose to discuss a book I'd recently read by John Diamond, *'C- because Cowards Get Cancer Too'*. It's a brutally honest account of John's battle with throat cancer and has been called funny, heart-breaking, un-put-downable and so re-readable, amongst other things. Interestingly though, it didn't go down well as a presentation. The reason? My colleagues felt utterly uncomfortable with even thinking about cancer, such is the power of the C word.

Cancer is indeed a word people dread. It conjures up images of aggressive treatment and, despite improvements in cancer mortality rates as expressed in percentage terms, is still a leading cause of death. As I write this the media have just announced the passing of TV personality Linda Bellingham, who had undergone over a year of treatment and surgery for colon cancer. So the treatments, despite all the hype and research dollars, don't always work.

Mainstream, first line cancer treatment falls into one of three categories – chemotherapy, radiotherapy and surgery. These treatments attack and often destroy the tumour, but with considerable collateral damage and a weakening of healthy cells too.

What if we were able to combine the power of the mainstream therapies with natural solutions that protect regular cells and help you to recover your underlying health, despite the aggressive treatment? Wouldn't that be something?

And what about recurrence? What if we can learn how to keep our bodies in a state of optimal health, so that we significantly increase the odds of remaining free from cancer once we have received the all clear? Is this indeed possible? Based on the dramatic improvements I experienced in my own health, and working extensively in healthcare over the last five years, I strongly believe that it is. A natural approach can also dramatically reduce your risk of developing cancer and other degenerative diseases in the first place.

If you are in any doubt about the power of natural therapies used alongside cancer treatment, I recommend a book called Radical Remission, by PhD researcher Dr Kelly Turner.[1] Within the cancer world there is something known as a spontaneous remission, where someone even with a terminal diagnosis makes a spectacular recovery. You might think that the medics would be pouring over these case studies, trying to understand anything that could be shared with others? Wrong! Dr Kelly found that although spontaneous remission was largely acknowledged in oncology, and many physicians had witnessed it first hand, there was no follow up or interest in discovering any contributing factors. Indeed some patients were asked not to discuss their own success so as not to raise 'false hopes'! Fortunately for us, Dr Kelly has made this her work, and is an inspiration to anyone affected by cancer either directly or through someone they love.

Dr Kelly identified that spontaneous remission is not spontaneous at all, but behind each and every person that had changed their diagnosis there is a whole stream of activities designed to improve their nutrition, emotional state, and social and spiritual connection.

Whether you are looking to increase your chances of outsmarting cancer or wanting to adopt a preventative approach in order to reduce the risk of developing a

chronic disease in the first place, this book will help you to focus on generating your own good health, naturally.

My Story

Like many people who change career direction and become involved in naturopathic health care, I have been at the receiving end of an unexpected and, at the time, very unwelcome diagnosis.

I was 39 years old and married with two small children. I was working part time in a management training company in a job I loved, and thought that it was well suited to family life. Often I'd work in the evenings, running training workshops and presentations sometimes up to two hours' drive from home. I'd set off around 4pm when my hubby arranged to come home from work, returning in the wee hours feeling quite hyped up. I would then crack through much of the admin associated with the job; I was that person sending emails at 3am! Obviously this curtailed my sleep somewhat, but with two young kids, I could always cat nap in the day.

We often associate stress with being in a negative situation, maybe with money worries, emotional turmoil, issues at home or work etc., but it really doesn't have to be. For those A type personality, adrenalin junkies out there, we can quite easily, and happily, generate our own stress which can be just as debilitating to how our bodies function. At the time, I would never have thought of myself as 'stressed', but on reflection I most certainly was.

As often goes hand in hand with a busy family and home life, I'd put on a bit of weight. At the time I thought I ate really well. Cereals for breakfast and lots (and lots!) of coffee. Cheese & onion toasties or sandwiches for lunch – my, was I fond of them! And a home cooked supper with the occasional glass of wine or two. So by most people's standards, fairly regular fayre and the type of diet the average doctor would think was fine. I often see food diaries like this, and it's not surprising really when we have crazy healthy eating guidelines which advocate up to 6-11 portions of starchy carbohydrates a day. We'll learn more about starches, or sugar, and cancer later.

Fortunately for me I was in the GP surgery in September 2003 with our daughter, reading a breast health poster in the waiting room. One thing struck me, which was that if there was any difference between the two breasts then you should see your doctor. I had some discomfort on the left side, and it was a little bit larger, which I'd just attributed to weight gain. There was also quite an obvious vein that wasn't on the other side, but of course I had no idea that tumours had the ability to grow their own blood vessels.

Anyway, to cut a long story short, I was referred on by the GP and subsequently diagnosed with grade 4 breast cancer. This was terrifying on many counts but particularly because the tumour was very large (11cm) and also the most aggressive grade, as it often is in younger women.

I don't think anyone could ever forget those words when they are delivered. I'm sorry Mrs Phillips but… We were absolutely shell shocked. My first thoughts went to our children, who were five and six years old at the time. The thought of not seeing them grow up was devastating.

The medical team, though, were brilliant. A nurse took us through the mammogram, pointing out the tumour (not hard to see) and 'calcification' seen as little white dots (calcium shouldn't be accumulating in our tissues!) The treatment plan was decided upon – chemotherapy, in an attempt to reduce the tumour size, and then surgery (known as neoadjuvant therapy).

At the same time, a work colleague was going through a similar experience with his wife and was also using naturopathic methods. He told me about the Penny Brohn Centre in Bristol, a world-renowned complementary therapy centre. This was our introduction into the complementary world, and a journey that I believe saved my life.

We all deal with personal crisis differently. For me, the default position is to read my way out of tricky situations. I started with *'Your Life in Your Hands'* by Jane Plant[2] and *'The Breast Cancer Prevention & Recovery Diet'* by Suzannah Olivier.[3] Their messages really resonated with me, and sparked a real interest in learning more about food as medicine, and lifestyle as health.

Given this new information, I started to re-engineer my diet and lifestyle. In a way I took my 'things to do list' and turned it upside down. Looking after myself suddenly became quite important! I took up yoga at home using a video to start with, then lessons, and eventually retrained as a yoga teacher. I learnt to meditate and even hugged trees. Reflexology was amazing during chemo; I can recall literally crawling in for a session several days after the first 'blast' of treatment and bouncing out an hour later. I addressed my working patterns and sleep.

But it was the food side of things that I really found fascinating. The thought that you can change your own biochemistry just by changing what you eat - wow! My new way of eating wasn't just good for me, but the food was totally delicious and very simple to organise too. I'll share this with you later. Later on I also took a lot of supplements, which were recommended by a nutritionist. I think these were very helpful to my recovery.

In terms of my cancer, the first round of chemo was brutal, and I was hospitalised for a week due to a potential infection and severe neutropenia, which is a very low white cell count. My white cells did not always recover quickly enough which on one occasion meant a delay to treatment of a few days. When you're all geared up to be 'poisoned' and people are involved to take care of you, this was really quite a blow. I was expecting a course of six treatments but after just three sessions the chemotherapy was deemed not to be working, in that the tumour size did not reduce. That was a difficult time.

I was offered a second opinion at the Royal Marsden and agreed to progress to surgery just before Christmas in 2003. All went well and, because the tumour cells had been well contained, radiotherapy was not necessary. So, January 2004 was a New Year and very much a New Me.

Since then I have easily and joyfully maintained this new lifestyle, and gone on to study for a Degree in Nutritional Medicine.

For the last 5 years, I've worked extensively with patients to help them regain optimal health, and am continually blown away by how effective this approach is. The pull to turn this knowledge towards cancer is now so great, that I have to share this information with you. I write this to inspire you, whatever your situation, to see through the commercialised world in which we live, and embrace a lifestyle in harmony with nature.

How to Use This Book

Eat to Outsmart Cancer has three sections.

Section One: (Chapters One and Two) strives to help you achieve a better understanding of cancer, and how cancer cells differ from regular cells. This knowledge will enable you to see the opportunities for making your internal terrain hostile to cancer cells and supportive of healthy, regular cells.

Although genetics plays a role in the development of cancer, it is hereditary in less than 10% of cases. Rather, in 90-95% of cases it is a complex interaction between our genes, our lifestyle, diet and the environment which causes cancer. The really good news is that there is, therefore, considerable scope to address our diet, lifestyle and environment both to reduce the risk of, and enhance recovery from, cancer.

Nutrition is especially important, because it provides the nutrients required to have a healthy, well-functioning, metabolically competent body. Yet most people are confused about how to eat well, and are seduced into short cuts by a powerful, profit-driven food industry.

Good nutrition is a powerful anti-cancer force. You can use it to strengthen your immune system and improve your ability to detoxify, thus efficiently removing chemicals and metabolites, which may corrupt your DNA. Learn how you can stack the odds against cancer cells by following an alkaline diet, avoiding sugar and oxygenating your body.

Section Two: (Chapters Three to Six) covers what you need to know to make healthy decisions around food. I set out the reasons why you need each of the macronutrients: fat, protein and carbohydrate. You can see that food is not just about calories. It also provides all of the raw materials for you to grow, replenish and function.

There are a number of controversies around any anti-cancer diet. Rather than you taking these at face value, I explore each in turn so that you can consider what is right for you.

There isn't necessarily one diet for everyone. The overriding goal is to focus on fresh, natural foods and strive for a balanced plate including protein, lots of vegetables, good fats, fruit and starch. This applies whether you have a varied diet (Mediterranean), are vegetarian (or vegan) or wish to avoid more inflammatory foods (paleo – no grains, dairy or pulses). The latter can be especially useful if your digestion is compromised.

Recipes are included to give you a head start in improving your diet, and also to reassure you that the meals produced in this way of eating really can be really delicious! Depending on your skill in the kitchen, you may like to supplement this book with a new cookbook, and several options are given in the Resources section.

Implementing a new diet does take extra thought and planning, but new, healthier habits can be quickly established. I give you tips on preparation, gadgets, sourcing, eating out and surviving on a budget. I also share some simple food preparation techniques to make life in the kitchen a breeze.

Section Three: (Chapters Seven and Eight) establishes a more personalised touch. Here I utilise a model of nutritional or functional medicine to consider health in the context of key biochemical processes – inflammation, digestion, stress, energy production and hormonal balance. Supplements and specific foods are considered to restore homeostasis or internal balance. The secret is to decide which elements may, or may not, be relevant to you, and consider working with a nutritional therapist if you think you might benefit from professional advice.

There are a number of very exciting biochemical tests available privately through a nutritional therapist or integrative doctor. These can be very helpful in establishing priorities and informing a personalised nutritional programme.

Your good health is one of the best investments you can make.

Chapter One: Cancer, We're Gonna Get You?

It is very tempting to think of cancer as something external to ourselves that can be destroyed and removed. Back in 1971, President Nixon launched the 'war against cancer' with the National Cancer Act in the US. This focused on increased research into drug therapies in an effort to find a cure for cancer. Yet here we are, over 40 years on, and cancer still poses a significant threat.

More recently, the National Cancer Institute in the USA approached Paul Davies, an eminent physicist, to take a completely fresh look at the science of cancer. Significant funding followed and 12 scientific centres have been set up specifically to study cancer biology. Davies is challenging conventional understanding and sees cancer, rather like ageing, as a condition that can be managed and its effects mitigated against[4].

This offers great hope for both prevention and recovery. If we understand the triggers which make the disease more likely to occur, then there is potentially scope to improve outcomes through dietary and lifestyle choices[5].

Why We Need Integrative Medicine

"Every two minutes in the UK, someone is diagnosed with cancer."
Cancer Research UK (2014)

The number of people affected by cancer is growing at an alarming rate. In 1975 the lifetime risk of developing cancer was around 25% or 1 in 4, yet latest estimates show that we are fast approaching 50% or 1 in 2.[6] The cancer charity, Macmillan, estimate that 2.5 million people in the UK are now living with cancer, an increase of almost half a million people compared to five years ago. Worryingly, 1 in 4 face ill health or disability post treatment.[7]

The most common cancers in women are breast (30%), lung (12%) and bowel (11%), whilst for men these are prostate (25%), lung (14%) and bowel (14%). Together these four account for over half of all newly diagnosed cancers. Cancer can develop at any age, although there is increased incidence in later years, with over a third of cancers being diagnosed in people aged over 75. Less than 2% occur in the under 24s.[8]

Every day 440 people in the UK lose their life to cancer. That's one person every four minutes. It's the second leading cause of death after heart disease, and is responsible for 162,000 deaths annually in the UK, and 8 million people worldwide. Only 50% of adult cancer patients are expected to survive 10 years or more.

How do we assess the cost of cancer? Within the UK, annual NHS costs for cancer services are £5 billion, but the cost to society as a whole – including costs for loss of productivity – are estimated to be in the region of £18.3 billion (2012/2013).[9] In terms of research, much of which is spent on drug development, investment is significant. In 2014 the charity Cancer Research UK (CRUK) spent £351 million on research, whilst the National Cancer Institute's budget exceeds $5 billion (2014).[10]

The personal costs also merit consideration. A diagnosis can tear families apart. It can deprive people of their ability to work and support themselves. Cancer and its subsequent treatment can cause debilitating side effects, some of which will persist. For example, patients may have ongoing issues with fatigue, weight gain, digestive problems or nerve damage. And what about the emotional side effects? Many people are able to make positive changes through their diagnosis and come out of it with better emotional health than they've had before, but others can be debilitated by the pain of their experience, or fear of a recurrence.

It is wonderful that we have organisations like the NHS and CRUK striving to cure cancer, and there have been many drug developments which save lives. However, I believe that the cancer industry, like most of our current healthcare system, doesn't adequately address the root causes of cancer and doesn't empower people to become part of their own health solution. As much as 75% of cancer is lifestyle related – including diet, smoking, obesity and alcohol.[11] Medical drugs cannot fix this.

The overriding medical viewpoint at the moment is that diet has nothing to do with cancer. I disagree. I believe that dietary and lifestyle changes can significantly help support recovery from cancer, and they can be used preventatively.

My own experience was to follow an integrative approach, combining medical treatment with a radical lifestyle overhaul. Along with significant changes to my diet, I also saw a nutritionist and took a lot of supplements. Although the first round of chemotherapy was difficult, looking after myself really helped with later rounds and I was even able to work part of the time. In fact, with the exception of spending a few days in bed each cycle, my energy was good and I felt really well. I'm sure this was thanks to my new regime which helped to negate the potential side effects of chemotherapy. I see this consistently now in practice, where good nutrition can make a huge difference to how well people are able to tolerate cancer treatment.

But it's not just about treatment either. Surely the higher goal should be to reduce the incidence of cancer, which is currently climbing at an alarming rate? We hear a lot about early detection and some drugs have been used prophylactically to reduce cancer risk, but these are not without side effects[12]. Addressing lifestyle issues has a huge capacity for prevention, potentially resulting in fewer people becoming a cancer statistic, and the only side effect being increased well-being. It's a real missed opportunity to ignore this.

Integrative medicine is emerging as a tour de force to bring together the best of both worlds – which is the undoubted power of medicine combined with diet, nutritional and lifestyle support. Learning more about how cancer forms will help to establish the benefits of such an approach.

What is Cancer?

Cancer is a complex disease, which is multi-factorial. By this I mean that there is rarely a single cause. Even with smoking, which is associated with a high risk of cancer, not everyone who smokes will develop cancer. There are a whole host of environmental and genetic influences which predispose an individual towards, or away from, a disease state. Learning more about the influencing factors in our environment that we can control, puts us in a much stronger position for managing our health long term.

The World Cancer Research Fund (WCRF) estimates that between 5-10% of cancers are caused directly from inheriting genes associated with cancer. 90- 95% are due to alterations or damage to the genetic material within cells and these are potentially modifiable.[13]

This is good news because it means that there is scope for us to influence recovery from, and prevention of, cancer, alongside medical treatment. I say this because once a cancer has been detected most people usually opt for swift and radical action – which may involve chemotherapy, radiotherapy and surgery. But alongside this, if we stop to consider what actions may strengthen our underlying health, we are in an all-around better position.

There is no pressure to make drastic changes to your lifestyle, or to feel stressed about what may have gone before. This way of thinking should open you up to a sense of empowerment, where you can make step changes towards regaining your health at your own pace. Keep a sense of perspective, and draw on those around you for support. There are only benefits to be obtained from treating your body in a way that means it is well nourished, gently exercised and emotionally sound.

How Do Cancer Cells Differ from Normal Cells?

Regular healthy cells know how to behave. They differentiate in order to fulfil a useful role in your body. Your cells all have the same genetic makeup, but what differs is how those genes are switched on or off in order to govern cell behaviour. This means that a liver cell is different to a heart cell, which in turn is different to a skin cell. In an adult, cell growth is controlled so that replication serves only to replace dead or damaged cells. Then, when a healthy cell is no longer able to do its job, it dies - a phenomenon known as apoptosis or cell suicide, which enables new cells to take its place. So your average, everyday cell lives in a very ordered way and contributes to the bigger picture of keeping you well.

Cancer cells are the rebels on the block. They have lost control of their normal growth and undergo uncontrolled replication. They may be less differentiated - this is what the tumour grade means. In general, tumours are graded between 1 and 4, depending on how abnormal they appear. The structure of grade 1 cells appears to be close to that of normal tissue, and these cells tend to be slow growing. In contrast, grade 3 and 4 cells are far less differentiated and tend to grow more rapidly.

Weinberg & Hanahan[14] have identified 6 hallmarks of cancer, which describe the way that cancer cells differ from regular cells:

1. Cancer cells induce and sustain growth-promoting signals, fuelling uncontrolled cell growth.

2. At the same time, they also circumvent efforts to regulate cell proliferation by evading growth suppressors.

3. They are resistant to cell death or apoptosis, giving a third mechanism by which cell proliferation can be maintained.

4. Whilst healthy cells undergo finite cell growth and division cycles, cancer cells exhibit unlimited potential to replicate – in essence they have immortality.

5. In order to sustain their own nutrient and oxygen supply, and evacuate metabolic waste, tumour cells induce angiogenesis, or the growth of new blood vessels.

6. They are able to invade the local tissue, and then spread or undergo metastasis to more distant locations and organs.

These changes happen progressively, and may take years or even decades to go from the initiation of the first cancer cells through to the detection of a solid tumour and on to metastasis. Each stage of that development presents an opportunity to change the environment within the body, and to make it increasingly hostile to cancer cells. Your diet and lifestyle are your biggest allies in protecting your health or supporting recovery from serious illness.

Fig 1: The Cancer Pathway

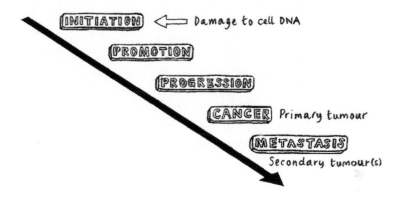

What Causes Cancer?

The WCRF has established a number of factors which are known to be causes of cancer.[15] These can be classified as those that are either developed from within (known as endogenous), and those that are derived from the external environment (exogenous). In reality, all of us produce some cells on a daily basis that have damaged DNA and thus the potential to cause cancer. But in a healthy body these are usually swiftly dealt with by the immune system. Cancer only takes hold when conditions are right for the damaged cells to proliferate and progress.

So let's now look at some of the initiators of DNA damage, which is the starting point for cancer initiation.

Internal Factors Contributing to Cancer Initiation:

1. Inherited Genetic Mutations

Just to re-iterate, a minority of cancers (5-10%) are linked to inherited genes. But what exactly is a gene? Located in your chromosomes, genes are like a recipe book with instructions to make the thousands of proteins which carry out very specific tasks in your body. A mutation refers to the equivalent of a mis-spelling or error in the recipe, resulting in a small, but sometimes significant change to the detailed structure of the resulting protein. Such mutations are referred to as a single nucleotide polymorphism (SNP). Many mutations are unimportant and have no negative impact on health. However, if the gene is essential and if the mutation affects how well its protein functions, then it can have dire health consequences.

In cancer, gene mutations can occur for the proteins which protect against tumour development, known as tumour suppressor genes. Examples include the BRCA1 and BRCA2 genes which are found in breast and other tissue. Another is the P53 gene. This is so important that it has been called the guardian of the genome. These genes produce proteins which provide protection by repairing or destroying damaged DNA. Individuals with tumour suppressor gene mutations are less efficient at this control, which can lead to an increased risk of developing cancer.

2. Oxidative Stress

Free radicals are all around us. We also produce them via our own metabolism, rather like a car produces exhaust fumes. But what are they, and what do they have to do with oxidative stress?

You may (or may not!) remember from your chemistry studies that molecules are made up of atoms which comprise protons, neutrons and electrons. When protons (positive charge) and electrons (negative charge) are in balance, then the molecule is stable, or electrically neutral. In contrast, free radicals have undergone a reaction, usually oxidation, which leaves them with at least one unpaired electron. This makes them highly reactive, in a quest to neutralise themselves. They aggressively attack other molecules in order to steal an electron, and this could include your own cells and DNA.

The body, though, has a defence mechanism. Antioxidants, which are widely available in natural foods and particularly vegetables, readily donate electrons and thus quench free radical activity. Vitamins A, C and E, selenium, and co-enzyme Q10 all have strong antioxidant properties, and are readily available as supplements.

Oxidative stress describes the damage that can ensue from high levels of free radical activity, either from increased exposure to oxidation, or insufficient dietary intake of antioxidants, or both. In our modern world, sources of oxidative stress are plentiful, including pesticides and toxins in the environment, foods such as sugar, alcohol, heat damaged oils and hydrogenated fats, radiation exposure and smoking. It can also be caused internally through stress, over exercise and inflammation.

A useful test for oxidative stress is urinary 8-hydroxydeoxyguanosine (8-OHdG), assessed as part of the Organic Acid Test described in Chapter Eight. 8-OHdG is one of the major products of DNA oxidation and a risk factor for cancer, atherosclerosis and diabetes. Elevated levels often correlate with hyperglycaemia indicating that high blood glucose can be a risk factor for oxidative stress. Elevated levels are also found in cancer patients[16]. For example, high levels of 8-OHdG are associated with a significantly shorter survival time in oesophageal cancer patients[17].

Reducing oxidative stress to protect yourself from DNA damage is important. One way to do this is to eat more antioxidant rich foods, particularly vegetables and fruits, including pomegranates, berries, spices, herbs, red kidney beans and apples. **This is why we need at least 5 a day...**

3. Inflammation

Inflammation is a physiological response to infection, irritation or trauma. It is the reason that swelling, redness and tenderness occur and it denotes the start of the healing process. So it is most definitely helpful in an acute context. Prolonged, chronic inflammation (where the acute inflammation fails to resolve) is, however, linked to both pain and chronic disease progression.

Chronically inflamed tissue is infiltrated with a variety of inflammatory cells which produce a wide variety of chemicals that can cause DNA damage and cancer promotion[18]. This can potentially predispose someone to cancer. For instance, people with an inflammatory condition known as Barrett's Oesophagus have a 125 times greater risk of developing oesophageal cancer compared with the general population. Approximately 5% of ulcerative colitis patients will go on to develop colon cancer.

Inflammation can also be insidious, smouldering from within, with very little in the way of active symptoms. Food intolerances, bacterial toxins (also gut related), infections or oxidative stress can be pathways to slow, gradual and repetitive injury to blood vessels, joints or tissue, causing low grade and continuous inflammation, which can eventually contribute to more serious pathology.

Evidence that inflammation is associated with cancer comes from a study of patients with invasive breast cancer. A seven-year study of breast cancer patients showed that those with elevated C reactive protein levels (CRP) – a blood marker for inflammation – had an increased risk of death. Five-year survival was 90% for those with lower CRP levels versus 74% for those in the higher range[19]. In other words, those with higher levels of inflammation had a 2.6 times greater increased risk of death.

Some foods can be a significant source of inflammation. In one study, individuals given a junk food, high fat, high carbohydrate meal experienced raised levels of an inflammatory marker (NF Kappa B) in their blood up to 3 hours after eating[20]. High glycaemic foods were also found to aggravate inflammatory markers in lean, young adults, and the authors conclude that this may help to explain relations between carbohydrates, glycaemic index, and the risk of chronic disease. This study showed that white bread induced the same inflammatory response as consuming sugar, and this was 3 times higher than after a pasta meal[21].

On the other hand, natural, whole and unprocessed foods and the nutrients they contain can reduce inflammation. In this book, I will be describing a diet that is based on this premise. One particularly potent supplement is curcumin, which is the active ingredient in turmeric. There are 2,664 references in the scientific journals for curcumin in relation to cancer, such is the interest in its therapeutic potential. Regularly using turmeric in spicy foods for instance is encouraged, and it is also an incredibly valuable supplement[22]. Aloe vera, omega 3 rich fish oils and antioxidants are also examples of supplements which reduce inflammation (more on this in Chapter Seven), along with rosemary, quercetin, vitamin D and olive leaf extract.

4. Hormones

Lifetime exposure to oestrogen is an established risk factor in female hormonally based cancers such as those of the breast, endometrium and ovaries. Contributing factors are thought to be early puberty, late menopause or not bearing children. Blood oestrogen levels prior to a cancer diagnosis are positively associated with breast cancer development. A meta-analysis of nine studies found that post-menopausal women with high blood oestrogen levels had roughly a twofold increase in breast cancer risk[23]. This risk is also relevant in pre-menopausal women.[24]

Making good food choices is an effective way to help balance hormone levels. The healthy metabolism and excretion of hormones requires well-functioning detoxification, and this is enhanced by vegetables from the cruciferous family (including broccoli, cauliflower, bok choy, cabbage and cress), onions, garlic, dark leafy greens such as kale and lemons. The second step of hormonal metabolism also requires ample amounts of B vitamins (particularly B6 and B12) and amino acids. There are many supplements which can help to support detoxification and these are discussed in Chapter Two.

In contrast, hormone levels tend to be higher in obese women, those who smoke and those who drink alcohol[25].

Genova Diagnostics offer a very helpful female hormone test panel which can identify individual blockages in hormone metabolism (see Chapter Eight). This identifies specific nutritional support required to restore hormonal homeostasis. There is more to come on this subject, and I will also discuss healthy hormone metabolism in Chapter Seven, which is about individualising your nutritional plan.

Environmental Factors

Carcinogenic substances are all around us, and the two ways of dealing with them are to limit exposure as much as possible, and to have a healthy detoxification capacity, so you can efficiently process and remove chemicals from your body. Key carcinogens include:

1. Tobacco

Tobacco causes an estimated 20% of all cancer deaths (and not just lung cancer) or 1.2 million deaths worldwide. Cigarette smoke contains at least 80 known carcinogens including arsenic, cadmium and formaldehyde. Smoke is also a source of oxidative stress. So if you are concerned about your health and still smoke – now is the time to give up.

It's worth noting here that lung cancer is not always caused by smoking – 20% of men and 50% of women with lung cancer are non-smokers.

2. Infectious Agents

Infectious agents including viruses, bacteria and parasites can induce DNA damage, increase inflammation and promote the development of cancer.

I'm sure you are aware that your gut is home to a considerable volume of microbes – many of which are friendly and essential for health, but some of which can be pathogenic (capable of causing disease). For example, the bacteria Helicobacter Pylori is the strongest known risk factor for gastric cancer[26]. Any pathogenic gut bacteria, or yeasts such as candida, will put a strain on your immune system, as they will produce toxic waste products which you then have to process. Having a robust gut is therefore imperative for maintaining good health.

In less developed countries, approximately 1 in 4 cancers are linked to infection, arising chiefly from inadequate nutrition.

3. Radiation

Both ionising radiation and ultra violet (UV) light have the potential to damage DNA and act as carcinogens.

Exposure to ionising radiation may often be unavoidable – sources include cosmic radiation which is present in the environment and originates from sources in space, natural radioactivity from rocks and soil, medical intervention such as X rays or atomic radiation from nuclear accidents (WCRF). Damage is induced either by causing breaks in DNA, or by generating free radicals. Your best protection may be to limit DNA damage from other modifiable sources and ensure a diet rich in antioxidants to reduce oxidative stress.

You can protect yourself from UV exposure from the sun by limiting access to direct sunlight, but there is a further consideration here. Vitamin D is produced by the action of sunlight on the skin, and this vitamin pays a significant role in cancer protection. So too rigorously avoiding the sun may not be good either. Whilst sun screen offers protection from the sun's rays, there has been some concern raised about potential carcinogenic compounds present in some brands[27]. So what do you do?

During the summer months enjoy limited exposure to direct sunlight for a short period, maybe 10- 20 minutes, but don't burn. When the sun is strong then either cover up or seek some shade. If you do use sunscreen, check the ingredients and seek a brand without parabens or oxybenzone. The use of tanning beds for cosmetic use is not recommended.

4. Industrial Chemicals

The wide scale use of a large number of chemicals and pesticides in food production is a very good reason to consider going organic. But what about the chemicals in your home, or the personal products and toiletries that you use? Find ways, where you can, to reduce your toxic load.

This might involve buying a steam cleaner rather than using chemicals, limiting your use of plastics or changing to more naturally based cosmetic and toiletry brands. I'm not going into detail of this here, but suffice to say, it is a very important issue. Two good organic ranges to consider are Defiant Beauty (www.jenniferyoung.co.uk) or Neal's Yard Remedies.

5. Carcinogens in Food

Keeping food as natural as possible is a good way to minimise your exposure to carcinogens in food. There are several potential sources:

You've probably heard that aggressive heat used in barbecuing over a direct flame can result in the production of carcinogenic compounds? These include heterocyclic amines and polycyclic aromatic hydrocarbons (PAH), which are formed by cooking meat at high temperatures. So keep cooking temperatures modest and absolutely avoid eating meats with charred surfaces. For everyday use, consider using a slow cooker, which is not only a healthy way to prepare meat (and pulses) but also scores very highly for convenience.

Processed meats often contain added nitrites and nitrates, used as preservatives, which can be converted to the carcinogenic N-nitroso compounds, either in the food, or once they have been eaten in the digestive tract. Having a healthy gut flora may be protective here, but it is good practice to eliminate or drastically reduce processed meats from your diet.

Acrylamides are a controversial by-product derived from heating starchy foods like crisps, French fries and cereal products to high temperatures. The International Agency for Research on Cancer considers acrylamide to be a "probable human carcinogen," based on studies in laboratory animals which were given acrylamide in their drinking water[28]. Despite this, there are currently no limits for acrylamide levels in food, and current research, whilst acknowledging the known DNA damage, concludes that the role of acrylamides in human cancer is unclear[29].

However for those of us who are quite keen to keep healthy, un-mutated DNA in our cells, it is prudent to avoid those foods known to be high in acrylamides. The good news is that these are exactly the highly processed foods that would be avoided on a health-giving, natural diet anyway.

Why is Nutrition Essential?

Despite the mounting evidence that our diet and lifestyles are driving the incidence of many chronic diseases, including cancer, the medical profession is still, by and large, fairly dismissive of the value of good nutrition and lifestyle modification alongside standard medical care (otherwise known as an integrative approach). Indeed current advice from a top London hospital actually discourages patients from eating fruit and vegetables and promotes the use of extra sugar, desserts and cake![30]

I strongly disagree with this advice, even in patients wanting to gain weight. As you will see later, vegetables are the most vital food group for health, providing a wealth of nutrients and fibre, whilst there is strong evidence that sugar actually feeds cancer cells (see Chapter Two).

The whole of this book supports the case that nutritional and lifestyle therapy are effective interventions both for cancer prevention and as an adjunct to medical treatment. In this section I'll highlight some information to reassure you that it really is worth the inconvenience of changing your diet and your lifestyle.

1. Diet is a leading cause of cancer.

The NHS Cancer Plan[31] states:

"After smoking, what people eat is the next biggest contributor to cancer deaths, and may be responsible for up to a third of all cancer deaths."

The World Cancer Research Fund[32] states:

"... cancer is 30 to 40% preventable over time, by appropriate food and nutrition, regular physical activity and avoidance of obesity. On a global scale this represents over 3 to 4 million cases of cancer that can be prevented in these ways, every year."

Also a review of 120 different research papers concludes that cancer is (largely) a preventable disease that requires major lifestyle changes[33]. This study finds that modifiable risk factors including diet, smoking, obesity and alcohol, may account for up to 75% of cancer cases.

Fig 2: Cancer risk factors

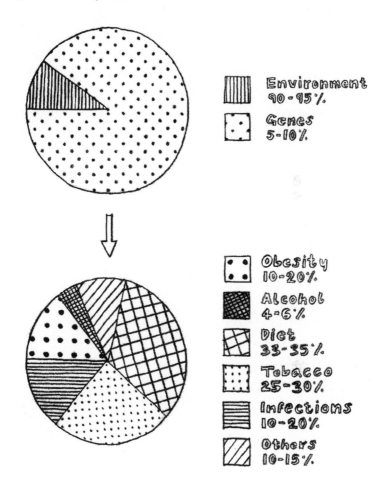

Environment
90-95%

Genes
5-10%

Obesity
10-20%

Alcohol
4-6%

Diet
33-35%

Tobacco
25-30%

Infections
10-20%

Others
10-15%

2. The inclusion of nutrient rich foods and a healthy lifestyle can slow and even inhibit cancer progression.

One particular study looked at the impact of intensive diet and lifestyle support on the progression of early stage prostate cancer.[34] The experimental group were given comprehensive advice and followed a real food diet with supplements, exercise, stress management and weekly support. The control group did not have access to additional advice or support, other than that generally offered by their physician.

Over the course of a year, the control group saw a gradual progression of their disease marked by increasing levels of Prostate Specific Antigen (PSA), whilst the experimental group had an overall reduction in PSA. Even more striking is the fact that the blood of those with diet and lifestyle support had an inhibitory effect on cancer cell growth. This test is known as LNCaP, and blood is applied to cancer cells in the laboratory. The experimental group showed an 8 fold greater inhibition of cancer cell activity versus those in the control group.

Fig 3: Study results from prostate cancer trial

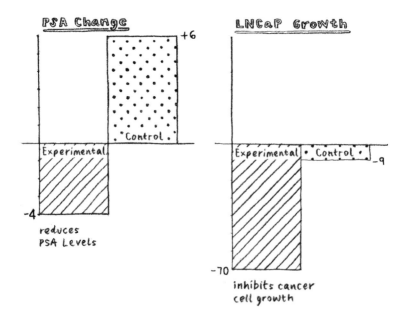

3. A growing body of people are using radical diet and lifestyle change to improve their prognosis, and even survive a terminal diagnosis.

High profile survivors include Kris Carr, who was diagnosed with a rare Stage 4 cancer affecting her lungs and liver in 2003. Her motto is 'make juice not war!'[35] In 2003, Chris Wark was diagnosed with Stage 3 colon cancer. He had surgery but refused chemo, instead turning to nutrition and natural therapies to help his body heal.[36] Chris is very active in the cancer community and his website *www.ChrisBeatCancer*.com contains lots of inspirational stories of people overcoming the odds to regain health.

I also mentioned Dr Kelly Turner, author of *Radical Remission*[37], in the introduction. Her PhD involved a year long trip around the world, visiting ten countries and interviewing 50 healers and 20 cancer survivors about their healing practices and techniques. Her research continued by interviewing over 100 radical remission survivors and studying over 1000 of these cases. She found that nutritional, spiritual and emotional therapies were widely utilised amongst people who had survived terminal diagnoses.

4. Real food nourishes a human body, which helps to protect and maintain good health.

There is no 'one size fits all' when it comes to nutrition, but there is one overriding caveat. That is, if you eat abundant natural foods, including plentiful portions of vegetables[38], your risk of chronic disease, including cancer, is reduced.

The Mediterranean diet[39], the paleo or caveman diet[40] and vegetarian / vegan diets[41] can all claim to be associated with lower rates of cancer. This should not be a surprise, as they share many of the same core principles, which are:

- A preference for using fresh ingredients rather than processed foods

- High consumption of vegetables and fruit

- Protein from either animal or plant based sources

- Liberal use of nuts and seeds

- Selection of unprocessed oils – for example olive oil and coconut oil

- Potential for a low refined sugar intake

Their differences may be a matter of personal taste, or it may be that some foods are excluded due to our biochemical differences. Indeed, the ideal diet for an individual may even vary throughout their lifetime. The Mediterranean diet features all of the main food groups and so offers the most scope, whilst a vegetarian diet excludes animal protein. (A vegan diet goes one stage further and excludes all animal products, even honey.)

The paleo diet is said to be based on the food availability of our ancestors. It excludes all grains, pulses and dairy and has proven very beneficial in cases of digestive issues and inflammatory conditions such as in Multiple Sclerosis. It is also popular for weight loss and retaining muscle mass (very important for healthy ageing).

The bottom line is – eating naturally is the best health choice you can make.

5. In contrast, typical western diets, which are high in processed and fast foods, result in reduced protection against disease.

A very interesting paper called '*Fast food fever*' reviews the impact of the Western diet on immunity[42]. It provides damning evidence against the over consumption of sugar, refined salt, saturated and omega 6 fats, and gluten – all of which are prevalent in processed foods. These have the potential to reduce immunity, yet increase inflammation, the hallmark of chronic diseases including cancer.

In addition, heavily processed diets often lack fresh fruits and vegetables, which provide the vitamins and minerals that are essential for optimal metabolic functioning. Bodies just don't work as efficiently without regular consumption of fresh produce.

6. Nutritional supplements provide additional therapeutic benefit when used judiciously.

When recovering optimal health, supplements can be very helpful to support individual requirements, alongside a good diet. Insufficiencies may arise because of poor absorption, insufficient dietary intake, or increased need.

Medications often cause nutritional insufficiencies. For example, commonly used ant-acid medications, including lansoprazole, cause vitamin B12 and magnesium deficiencies[43].

Chemotherapy drugs also cause nutritional deficiencies[44] and this may contribute to some of their side effects. Despite the unwillingness of many oncologists to support the use of supplements, two reviews of the clinical evidence have shown that supplements used alongside chemotherapy can increase the effect of chemotherapy, reduce side effects and protect normal tissue. Both also report increased survival rates.[45] [46]

Hopefully you can now see how important good nutrition is to your health in respect of cancer risk. It is important to take this information on board as a source of opportunity, and not as a criticism of any previous choices. We live in a toxic food environment, where unhealthy foods are persistently promoted. It's sometimes hard not to be taken in by them and the convenience they offer.

Government health guidelines are also not beyond reproach. An article in the New York Times discusses the severe limitations of the observational studies which have been used to define public health policies.[47] It's becoming increasingly apparent that some of the official advice could be misleading, or even harmful.

What you need now is to learn how to make better food and lifestyle choices, to give yourself the best health possible. And remember:

Looking after yourself is not a luxury, it's essential to a long and happy life.

Chapter Two: Nutrition as an Anti-Cancer Strategy

Now that you understand a little about how cancer forms in the body, let's turn our attention to creating the conditions which may help to actively prevent cancer cells establishing themselves and proliferating. This is relevant whether you are looking to prevent cancer, are currently having treatment, or are striving to avoid a re-occurrence.

Firstly, you need to build a strong immune system. This is because in everyday life we all make abnormal cells with DNA damage that have the potential to become cancerous, but our immune system seeks them out and destroys them. So a well-functioning immune system is the first line of defence against cancer.

Secondly, we'll look at how you can utilise your diet and lifestyle to stack the odds against cancer cells. You will learn that cancer thrives well in an acidic environment, loves sugar and hates oxygen. Your role then is to do just the opposite. Focus on alkaline foods, avoid sugar and breathe!

Finally, I will review the process of detoxification so that you are equipped with some inexpensive and easy strategies to reduce your toxic load.

Building a Strong Immune System

Think of your immune system as your very own army, on surveillance 24/7. Its aim is to protect you by effectively dealing with bacteria, viruses and other unwelcome visitors. The relative strength of an immune system is why one person may succumb to an infection, whilst another in the same household, exposed to the same germs, will not be affected.

An indication of a healthy immune system is a fast and efficient recovery from an infection, such as a cold. In contrast, an immune system that is overloaded may be sluggish, and the feeling of being below par may be fairly constant or frequent, with a slow resolution of symptoms. This can arise when the immune system is overwhelmed with an ongoing low grade infection, which is perpetrating an inflammatory response.

From a cancer point of view, we all produce cells with genetic mutations in our bodies every single day. The immune system plays a critical role in clearing such cells so as to prevent the development of cancer. Let's look at some of the ways in which you can support your immune system using nutrition.

If you are going through cancer therapy, then always discuss supplement regimes with your oncologist and consider working with a nutritionist or functional medicine practitioner to ensure compatibility with treatment.

Probiotics and Gut Health

The digestive system has the largest surface area of your body which is in contact with the outside world. Whilst previously estimated to equate to the surface area of a tennis court, this has recently been revised to an area of 30-40 square metres, or about half the size of a badminton court, which is still a very large area![48] 70-80% of our immune cells are located in the gut, where they are protecting the most significant point of entry into the body.[49] This means that gut health and immune health are intrinsically linked.

An imbalance of many types of gut bacteria creates a serious challenge for the immune system. Probiotics are the good bacteria which live symbiotically within our internal ecosystem where we provide nourishment in return for their activity. From an immune point of view, our microflora produce nutrients, such as butyrate, which keep the intestinal cells healthy. This helps to maintain tight junctions between the cells and keep pathogens and undigested food out of the bloodstream.[50] In sufficient quantities they strive to keep pathogenic bacteria, yeasts and parasites at bay. The latter can generate carcinogens and tumour promoting substances including secondary bile acids and heterocyclic amines.[51] Improving the gut flora also leads to reduced systemic inflammation[52], which is a significant driver for cancer.

If you suffer from any gut related problems such as acid reflux, constipation, diarrhoea, gas or bloating then this is a problem on two levels. Inefficient digestion means that you will not get the full goodness from your food, no matter how good your diet is. But just as importantly, if you are harbouring gut pathogens, this potentially has a significant effect on your immune system, adding to systemic inflammation and increasing your toxic load.

There are many challenges to our gut bacteria in the modern world we inhabit, for instance, from processed foods, antibiotics and other medications, alcohol and sugar. The *Outsmart Cancer* eating plan will steer clear of many of these, but it can still be helpful to boost probiotic levels, either through fermented foods on an ongoing basis (See Chapter Six), or by taking a course of high quality probiotics.

Probiotics have been found to be safe and beneficial to use alongside cancer treatment. In a randomised control study, patients receiving 5-Fluorouracil (5-FU) based chemotherapy and probiotic supplementation experienced reduced frequency of severe diarrhoea, reported less abdominal discomfort, needed less hospital care and had fewer chemotherapy dose reductions due to bowel toxicity.[53]In a further study, probiotic lactic acid-producing bacteria were found to be an easy, safe, and feasible approach to protect cancer patients against the risk of radiation-induced diarrhoea.[54]

Vitamin C

Vitamin C is probably one of the most well-known immune supportive nutrients, and for good reason.

Humans are one of the few mammals that can't make their own vitamin C, and so we have to get it from the food that we eat. It's widely available in fruits and vegetables, but unfortunately only 1 in 5 Britons eat even the recommended '5 a day'.[55] Vitamin C is a powerful antioxidant which protects cells from oxidative stress. It is essential for the development of connective tissue, wound healing and a number of metabolic functions, including the activation of folic acid, conversion of cholesterol to bile acids and production of the happy hormone, serotonin. Vitamin C protects the immune system and fights off infection.[56]

Vitamin C's role in cancer management has been controversial since the 1970s when Linus Pauling, an American chemist and twice Nobel prize winner, strongly advocated Vitamin C for maintaining health. He first published *Vitamin C and the common cold* in 1970, followed by *Cancer and vitamin C*. In 1976 he published the results of a study with Ewan Cameron, a cancer surgeon. They gave vitamin C therapy to 100 terminal cancer patients and compared their outcome to 1000 patients receiving conventional therapy only. Mean survival time was 4.2 times greater in the vitamin C cohort (210 days versus 50 days) and, importantly, 10% of the test subjects achieved survival averaging 20x that of controls.[57]

A recent animal study suggests that vitamin C helps to maintain the activity of your Natural Killer (NK) cells. These are immune cells which are especially fast to react against viruses and tumor cells. Mice supplemented with vitamin C had greater immune activity and survival rates.[58]

Ensuring a high intake of vegetables and modest fruit consumption is beneficial for lots of nutritional reasons including access to vitamin C. Excellent sources include peppers, watercress, broccoli, cabbages, berries and lemons. If you are eating well and in good health, then supplementation at times, for instance if you have a cold, can be helpful. If you are working to regain health, then vitamin C supplementation can be very useful at levels of 1 - 2g per day.

It is also possible to access high dose intravenous vitamin C (IVC) therapy privately. There are studies which suggest it can kill cancer cells and may make chemotherapy more effective.[59] There are also documented benefits about significantly reducing the side effects of cancer treatment, including fatigue, nausea, insomnia, constipation and depression. One study, involving newly diagnosed stage III-IV ovarian cancer patients, reported half of the adverse events compared to the control group when treated with IVC alongside chemotherapy.[60]

Vitamin D

This essential vitamin is actually a group of steroid hormones synthesized from cholesterol by the action of sunshine on the skin. It is also present in some foods (dairy, fish and eggs). It is very common to have a vitamin D insufficiency, or levels that are below an optimal range. One study of club level athletes showed deficiency levels of 57%[61], whilst for a group of breast cancer patients, 76% were deficient at diagnosis and those with lower levels had less favorable outcomes.[62] Indoor living, covering up and sun screens probably all contribute to a lack of sun induced levels of vitamin D.

Vitamin D is best known for its contribution to bone health and calcium metabolism. However it has a much wider role than that.

Most cells, including those of the immune system, have vitamin D receptors which regulate the expression of more than 200 genes responsible for cell differentiation, proliferation and programmed cell death (apoptosis), which is exactly the type of cellular activity to protect us from cancer.

Vitamin D also plays a role in gut health, where it is protective of the mucosal barrier of the digestive tract and hence helps to prevent pathogens and large food proteins from entering the blood steam. This was apparent in vitamin D deficient mice exposed to infection, which showed an increased intestinal permeability and an altered composition of gut bacteria versus controls. [63]

Vitamin D can easily be supplemented, but you may prefer to run a test to determine the dosage for you. As a fat soluble vitamin it is not easily excreted from the body and hence could potentially build up to toxic levels, contributing to issues with calcium metabolism, kidney stones and bone demineralisation. This can be done as a simple home test (blood spot) for around £30.

The definition of deficiency is 25 nmol/L or below, but optimal levels are regarded to be 75 – 200nmol/L. At very low levels, dosing may be up to 50,000 IU per week for 6 weeks and then retest.[64] When required, up to 2,000IU daily is a maintenance dose, along with a healthy calcium intake (dairy, green leafy veg, nuts, seeds).

Medicinal Mushrooms

Medicinal mushrooms are widely used alongside conventional cancer therapies in Asia, due to their immune supportive effects.

Martin Powell is a Chinese herbalist, biochemist and authority on medicinal mushrooms[65]. He explains that our immune system evolved alongside fungal pathogens and hence is able to recognise the structure of the mushroom cell wall as foreign. The long carbohydrate chains, or polysaccharides within mushrooms bind to immune receptors and help to balance the immune system, up-regulating when you need to fight infection, and down-regulating the inflammatory response. This includes:

- Activation of immune cells, including NK cells

- Increased antibody production

- Increased immune activity against a range of cancers

- Inhibition of tumour metastasis

Mushrooms very often get bad press in health circles, as there is a belief that they promote candida, or other fungal infection. However, the research doesn't back this up, and Martin reassures us that this, in his opinion, is completely untrue. In contrast, mushrooms have traditionally been used to treat candida related conditions and may be an ideal choice because:

- They don't contain the simple sugars that stimulate candida growth

- They increase the effectiveness of the immune response to candida and other fungi

- They are a rich source of anti-fungals. Just as animals in the wild compete for food, so do mushrooms, and hence they have evolved a range of anti-fungal compounds to gain advantage

There are many types of medicinal mushroom. The oriental types include shitake and oyster mushrooms, amongst others. These are widely available in either fresh or dried form and can be used generally in immune boosting recipes. Even regular button mushrooms have some anti-cancer properties.[66] With active cancer, or when in recovery, supplements may also be considered.

Coriolus is the most widely researched of all the medicinal mushrooms. The coriolus extracts, PSK and PSP show extended 5 year survival in many types of cancer, significantly boosted immune cell production, improved quality of life and reduced pain. They have good tolerability and are also compatible with cancer treatments.[67]

Reishi also has an established track record with respect to cancer. In prostate cells it has been shown to inhibit proliferation and induce apoptosis.[68] In addition to polysaccharides, Reishi contains triterpenoids, which have been reported to possess many anti-tumour benefits, including discouraging the growth of blood vessels to supply cancer cells (anti-angiogensis).[69]

So eat up your mushrooms and consider supplementing if your immune system is in need of support.

Polyphenols

Polyphenols are bioactive compounds that occur naturally in certain foods and drinks. They provide colour and flavour, and so the advice to 'eat a rainbow' is a sure way to include lots of these foods in your diet. They occur naturally in tea, coffee, red wine, chocolate, olives, olive oil, onions, herbs and spices, and also fruits, including apples and pomegranates.

Numerous studies have attributed polyphenols with a wide range of biological activity, including anti-inflammatory, antioxidant, cardiovascular protective and anti-cancer properties. They also play a significant role in immune function.[70]

Some examples are below, and of course there are many others:

Green Tea: Consumption of green tea has been associated with an improved prognosis in breast cancer patients, including a decreased risk of recurrence. The active ingredient in green tea is epigallocatechin gallate (ECGC). In an in vitro study of highly aggressive inflammatory breast cancer cells, EGCG decreased the expression of the genes that promote proliferation, migration, invasion, and survival. Clinical trials have also demonstrated efficacy of green tea polyphenol extracts in treatment of prostate cancer and leukaemia.[71] Two to three cups daily is ideal.

Curcumin: This is the active ingredient in the yellow Indian spice Turmeric and, as already mentioned, is being actively studied for its anti-inflammatory and anti-cancer potential. It is frequently used in Indian cookery and is a very good reason to enjoy a homemade curry. At therapeutic levels (4g daily) one study shows the potential of curcumin to slow progression in multiple myeloma.[72] Absorption can be an issue and many supplements are formulated to overcome this. Look for those that also contain piperine or black pepper. Curcumin is also suitable for use alongside cancer treatments and can help to reduce the side effects of chemotherapy and radiotherapy.[73]

Pomegranate Extract: This has been studied particularly in prostate cancer. A Phase ll study has shown a significant increase in the Prostate Specific Antigen doubling time (indicating a slower disease progression) with pomegranate extract.[74]

Professor Robert Thomas, Consultant Oncologist at Bedford and Cambridge University Hospitals and author of '*Your Lifestyle after Cancer*'[75], has combined the three polyphenols above with broccoli extract (which promotes detoxification) in a supplement called Pomi-T. Early clinical trials, again in prostate cancer, showed a significantly lower increase in the prostate tumour marker PSA in the group taking Pomi-T supplements. Whilst this group saw an increase in PSA of 15%, those without supplementation saw PSA increases of 78%. Pomi-T slowed the progression of PSA by more than five times.[76]

The *Outsmart Cancer* Diet encourages you to focus on fresh, natural ingredients, including lots of colourful fruits and vegetables to ensure that you consume lots of polyphenols.

Stack the Odds Against Cancer Cells

An Alkaline Diet

The most beneficial thing about an alkaline diet is that you consume whole, non-processed, natural foods which are teaming with nutrients.

You may remember the whole concept of acid and alkali, or pH, from school days. pH is a measure of the hydrogen ion (H+) concentration in a solution on a scale of 0- 14, where:

> 0-7 is acid (more H+ ions)
>
> 7 is neutral (distilled water)
>
> 7-14 is alkaline (less H+ ions)

It is important to acknowledge that the pH of your blood remains held in a very tight range of 7.36 − 7.44. However it is the fluid around your cells, called the interstitial fluid, which fluctuates depending on your metabolism and diet.

If you have ever kept fish, this concept will be familiar to you. Imagine that the fish are the cells in your body and the water is the interstitial fluid. Any keen aquarium owner will know that the pH of the water must be monitored − if it becomes too acidic the fish will die. The acidity comes from the waste products of the fish, in the same way that your cells produce waste products from their activity.

You may have heard that 'cancer loves an acidic body' and indeed there is research to show that acidity promotes the growth of cancer cells.[77]. This may be because cancer cells produce lactic acid as a by-product of their own metabolism. They make energy via the anaerobic fermentation of sugar (also known as glycolysis[78]), which regular cells only default to in times of inadequate oxygen availability. (Ever had aching muscles after heavy exercise and commented on a 'lactic acid build up'?)

Regular cells have a considerably more efficient means of energy production using oxygen and therefore don't usually need to use this pathway. However, if regular cell metabolism becomes compromised, by having insufficient nutrients, or damage to the mitochondria (the energy generators of the cell), then they too can revert to glycolysis and increase acidity through lactic acid production. A lack of B vitamins, magnesium, iron and amino acids will impair normal energy production, as will exposure to heavy metals, such as mercury, fluoride, aluminium and arsenic.[79] More about this when you learn about boosting your metabolism in Chapter Seven.

How else would your body become acidic? Just like the fish in acidic water, poor management of metabolic waste is a likely cause. Contributing factors can be excessive exposure to toxins, impaired detoxification (see later in this section), and poor lymph circulation (which transports waste products from the cells to the liver for processing).

Diet also plays a role in maintaining your acid alkaline balance.

Applying Alkaline to Your Diet

When foods are digested, they give rise to molecules which contribute to the acidity or alkalinity of interstitial fluids. So it's not about the acidity of the food before ingestion, but the resulting molecules arising from digestion. Vinegar and lemons are alkalising, because they are nutrient rich.

Foods rich in the minerals sodium, potassium, calcium and magnesium are alkaline. Plant based products score very highly here. Foods containing lots of nitrogen, sulphur, phosphorus and chlorine are more acid forming.[80] These include high protein foods and animal products. Processed foods are acid forming due to a low content of alkalising minerals. Alcohol depletes you of alkalising magnesium (and other nutrients) which are required for detoxification.

Alkaline Foods	Acidic Foods
All vegetables, especially leafy greens	Meat
Sprouted beans	Dairy
Lentils	Eggs
Almonds	Alcohol
Lemons & Limes	Processed foods
Quinoa	Fizzy drinks
	Wheat
	Rice

Foods abundant in vitamins and minerals (natural foods!) provide the co-factors necessary to ensure a strong metabolism which produces aerobic energy over glycolysis (minimising lactic acid) and detoxifies waste efficiently (keeping the fluids free from acidic waste). To me this is even more important than the individual effect of various foods.

Hence, I propose that an alkaline diet is one which is abundant in nutrient rich whole foods – including lots of vegetables and some fruit. It should also include moderate amounts of protein and this may be from both animal and plant based sources such as meat, fish, nuts, seeds, pulses and possibly a little dairy (from goats or sheep).

Some people may interpret an alkaline diet as vegan, arguing that animal products are "too acidic". However, animal products are also nutrient dense, and a very rich source of methionine, a sulphur containing amino acid which is a precursor to glutathione, your most important detoxification enzyme. I do think that it is all about balance, and keeping the 'nutrient rich' mantra in mind will lead you to a small steak with a big salad and not a burger in a bun (acidic) with chips and cola (also acidic).

There may be times when a 100% plant based diet is appropriate, however in my opinion there may be issues with excluding animal products long term, unless you are very judicious about ensuring sufficient protein and vitamin B12 intake (see Chapter Three).

Sugar - The Bitter Truth

For the last 5 decades, fat has taken the rap almost single-handedly for its alleged role in contributing to ill health and weight gain. I frequently meet people who are convinced that they are eating healthily because they are on a low fat diet. But the facts beg to differ.

In 2009 Robert Lustig, a Professor of Clinical Pediatrics and an endocrinologist at the University of California, challenged the dominant thinking about food and health when he delivered a lecture called 'Sugar: the bitter truth'. Posted on YouTube, this lecture went viral and made a strong case that it is sugar, not fat, that is driving the obesity epidemic through its deleterious effects on insulin signalling.[81] Insulin is the hormone which manages your blood sugar levels.

In 2013 Lustig visited the UK for a series of speaking engagements and fuelled the start of the backlash against the anti-fat mantra. Since then, 'fat doesn't make you fat' headlines abound, and the public are waking up to sugar as the real villain. We're startled to hear that hidden sugar is in many favourite foods, and that 'a bowl of tomato soup or vanilla yoghurt has as much sugar as a bowl of Frosties'.[82] The important thing to note here is that ALL carbohydrates are broken down into sugar (glucose) during digestion. This is why foods we don't necessarily perceive to be sweet, like bread, potatoes or canned tomato soup, are also a significant source of sugar.

The question is does sugar have anything to do with cancer? Yes. Indeed, it does.

Tumours consume significantly more sugar than do normal healthy tissues in order to sustain their growth. Researchers at UCL in London have used this information to revolutionise MRI scanning for detecting cancer. The sugar content equivalent of just half a regular bar of chocolate is sufficient to make tumours 'light up' in an MRI scanner and enables a safe and simple method to image tumours in detail. Great for use in a clinical situation, but what if you eat half a bar of chocolate every day?

No tumours would light up outside of an MRI, but they would be very happily guzzling sugar to fuel their own needs.[83]

This gives us a vital clue to a potential role of sugar in cancer growth and there are many studies that support this. One trial looked at the activity of tumour cell cultures exposed to normal glucose concentrations (5.5mM) compared to levels associated with poor glucose control (11mM). Higher glucose levels are associated with an altered expression of genes that promote cell proliferation, migration and adhesion of tumour cells. When insulin was added to the high glucose medium, proliferation rates were increased by up to 40%.[84] Insulin is the hormone involved in blood sugar regulation. It helps glucose to enter cells where it can be utilised as energy; in this case, it is probable that the insulin was helping to move glucose into the cancer cells, thus fuelling growth.

Moving on to animal studies, a low carbohydrate, high protein diet has been found to slow tumour growth and, just as importantly, to prevent cancer initiation in the first place. (Remember that carbohydrates are a source of blood glucose or sugar.) Tumour-bearing mice were fed equal calories made up from either a low carbohydrate diet, or a Western diet (high carb, low protein). Only one mouse on the Western diet achieved a full life span, whilst more than 50% of the low carbers reached or exceeded their normal lifespan. The low carb-fed mice had better glucose control, insulin and lactate levels. (Lactate is the acid produced by glycolysis, the favoured metabolic pathway of cancer cells.) Cancer initiation was also studied in mice genetically engineered to have an elevated risk of cancer. 50% of the mice on the Western diet had tumours within one year whereas none of the low carb mice were affected. This gives strong evidence that cancer flourishes on a high carbohydrate diet, which makes perfect sense from a physiological point of view. Cancer cells flourish in a sugar-rich environment.[85]

So what do human trials tell us about the relationship between a high carbohydrate (sugar) diet and cancer? Prospective studies are a commonly used methodology for dietary based research. A group (cohort) of subjects is recruited without any signs of disease, and followed for a period of time, usually several years. This can yield rich information about associations between risk factors and disease outcome.

Such a study was conducted in France with postmenopausal women looking at the risk of breast cancer. Of 62,739 women recruited and followed for 9 years, 1812 cases of breast cancer were recorded. This particular study was looking for any association between cancer incidence and carbohydrate intake. What it found was that, with women of normal weight (BMI <25), there was no established link with carbohydrate intake. But for heavier women (BMI>25), and those with a large waist circumference, there was a statistically significant association between rapidly absorbed carbohydrates and postmenopausal breast cancer risk.[86]

The European Prospective Investigation into Cancer & Nutrition (EPIC) study is one of the largest cohort studies in the world with over half a million participants recruited across 10 European countries and followed for almost 15 years. The Italian section comprised 26,066 women who were studied for 11 years and 879 were diagnosed with breast cancer during the period. This prospective study found that in a Mediterranean population which typically has a high and varied carbohydrate intake, a diet high in sugars and refined carbohydrates (with a high glycaemic load) plays a role in the development of breast cancer.[87]

Hence, we can conclude that high blood sugar levels (from consuming fast releasing or refined carbohydrates) create conditions which encourage cancer. Susceptibility also plays a role. Therefore in order to protect yourself against cancer, or to facilitate recovery, the solution must be to focus on foods which maintain steady levels of blood sugars. I will describe these foods in more detail in Chapter Four.

Dr Xandria Williams, author of *Vital Signs for Cancer*[88], has a wonderful way of illustrating this point. She says to imagine that your cells are like beggars, begging for food or glucose. The healthy cells have a small bowl and the cancer cells, who need so much more fuel relatively speaking, have a huge bowl. With limited glucose in the blood stream everyone gets some glucose. But when there's a huge surge in glucose, from eating fast releasing or refined carbohydrates, then the cancer cells, by virtue of their big bowls, prosper and meet their needs to fuel growth. In essence, a high sugar diet feeds cancer cells.

Oxygen

The ability of cancer cells to satisfy their energy requirements by glycolysis enables them to survive and thrive in low oxygen environments. Normal blood oxygen saturation is 95 – 100% and strategies to optimise your oxygen saturation and circulation form part of an anti-cancer strategy.

Haemoglobin in your red blood cells transports oxygen to the tissues. If you have a blood test from your doctor this will usually include a measure of your haemoglobin and it is worth knowing your levels. An optimal range for men is 125- 170 g/L and for women 115 – 150g/L.[89] Low levels may indicate anaemia – in which case your iron and ferritin levels should be checked; ferritin is the storage form of iron. Food sources of iron are red meat, particularly liver. Only supplement with iron if lab results indicate a deficiency. Select an organic form which is bioavailable and easily absorbed, such as iron bisglycinate. Also ensure an adequate intake of vitamins B12 and folate, which are used in the production of red blood cells. Food sources include sardines, liver, eggs and spinach.

The MacMillan Cancer Support report *'Move More – physical activity the underrated wonder drug'* highlights the benefits of exercise for both cancer recovery and prevention.[90] Gentle exercise, which can be as little as a short walk three times a week, can help to reduce tiredness and make you feel more alive. Exercise increases your heart rate and circulation, potentially resulting in increased oxygen flow to the tissues.

Deep breathing can also be helpful. When we're rushed or stressed our breathing can become shallow, often using just the top third of the lungs. So take time during the day to sit still, focus on long, steady deep breaths and feel that you are filling up on oxygen. Incorporating meditation into your day is a really good way to achieve this.

Nutritional Approaches to Support Detoxification and Elimination

Toxic compounds result from your body's own biochemical processes (rather like the exhaust of a car), or from the breakdown products of medications. They can be ingested with our food and drinks, or absorbed through the skin from the chemicals that are all around us. An unhealthy gut can also contribute to your toxic load from the waste products of pathogenic bacteria and yeasts.

Toxins have the potential to cause DNA damage, and hence require priority treatment to nullify their harmful effects and either excrete them, or store them out of harm's way. For example, Bisphenol A (BPA), which is widely used in plastics manufacture, has been shown to cause DNA strand breaks and damage in proteins, including those of the tumour suppressor gene P53.[91]

The main organs of detoxification are the kidneys and the liver, which process unwanted waste products into safe metabolites for removal via the urine or stool. The skin and lungs also participate in toxin removal through sweating and breathing.

The liver plays a key role in the biotransformation of toxic compounds into less harmful forms prior to excretion. This is just one of the many roles it plays, and the more you learn about natural wellness, the more you will come to realise that loving your liver is a cornerstone of good health. Residual toxins are by definition fat-soluble, otherwise they would already have been excreted via the urine. A two stage detoxification process first transforms the toxin into a water soluble molecule and then conjugates or adds a further molecule to escort it out of the body. Once transformed, the exit route is via the bile and into the intestine for excretion.

Phase 1 detoxification is catalysed by a family of enzymes known collectively as cytochrome P450. This first stage results in free radical production and so requires an abundance of antioxidants to quench their activity. These are found in a wide range of fresh foods, including:

Vitamin A – carrots, liver, watercress

Vitamin C – peppers, watercress, broccoli

Vitamin E – seeds, sardines, salmon

Selenium – nuts and seeds - particularly brazil nuts

This is followed by Phase 2 activity, and there are a number of pathways that can be utilised. Glutathione is an amino acid and powerful antioxidant involved in phase 2. It is derived from the amino acid cysteine, which is found in cruciferous vegetables (cabbage, kale, sprouts, broccoli, cauliflower etc.). Cruciferous vegetables are also a source of indole-3-carbinol, which is a powerful detoxifier of hormones. B vitamins (particularly B12, B6 and folic acid) support an important biochemical process called methylation, and are also essential. High homocysteine levels (measured in blood or via urine) can indicate a lack of these vital nutrients. Sulphur from eggs, onions and garlic provide the raw materials for the sulfation detoxification pathway. So you can see how important it is to have a varied and vegetable rich diet.

Having a well-functioning detoxification system is vital to good health and taking steps to strengthen removal of toxic and inflammatory molecules is essential in health recovery.

Detox Techniques

In addition to supporting liver function through nutrition, there are things that you can do at home, as part of your own self-care, to facilitate detoxification and elimination. These are easy to do and take very little in the way of resources. They also allow you some positive time to consciously focus on your own health, which can only be a good thing.

There are some inexpensive pieces of equipment you may consider investing in, and suppliers are listed in the Resources section.

1. Dry Skin Brushing

The skin is a major organ of elimination, and waste products are discharged through its surface on a daily basis. If the skin becomes less active at doing this, then it places an increasing burden on the kidneys and liver, which then have to compensate.

Stimulating the skin through dry skin brushing can help to mobilise and speed up the release of toxins. Circulation is improved and the lymphatic system is activated, thus moving waste from storage deep inside the tissues to the liver and kidneys for processing and excretion.

What you need:

A soft body brush with a long handle

How to do it:

Begin with dry skin before bathing or showering. Starting at the soles of the feet, make strong, short, and circular brush strokes travelling up the legs. Then move over your abdomen and back, always moving in the direction of the heart. Lastly work on the hands and arms. All in all, you should be done in around 5 minutes. A great way to set you up for the day!

2. Saunas

Another good technique which stimulates lymphatic flow and circulation to encourage the removal of cellular waste is spending some time in a sauna. The steam and high temperature cause perspiration, so ensure that you drink plenty of water to flush the impurities through. Taking saunas is also relaxing and refreshing for the mind and spirit. Infra-red saunas are the most effective for detoxification.[92]

3. Epsom Salt Baths

This is an easy one – place half a cupful of Epsom salts (magnesium sulphate) and a few drops of lavender oil in a bath and relax!

Why? Both magnesium and sulphate are easily absorbed through the skin. Magnesium is one of the four most important minerals in the human body. It helps regulate hundreds of enzymes and is involved in muscle control, detoxification, electrical impulses and energy production. Our preoccupation with calcium (which is rarely deficient) can also upset the balance with magnesium, as these two vitally important minerals work as a pair. Calcium is the 'hardening' mineral (and a high intake is linked with heart disease in females), whilst magnesium is the gentle, relaxing mineral.

Sulphate plays a key role in brain health, joints and the integrity of the digestive tract. It is also part of certain detoxification pathways. Epsom salts can be found in pharmacies or online.

4. Oil Pulling

This is an ancient Ayurvedic therapy which improves the overall health of the mouth, but may also have far wider benefits. Periodontal or gum disease is known to be a source of chronic inflammation, and is a risk factor for coronary heart disease.[93] Poor oral health is also associated with cancer, again it is inflammation that can be a trigger[94], and periodontal treatment significantly improves outcome for many cancers.[95] Hence, regular visits to the dentist should be encouraged, together with effective oral hygiene at home.

Oil pulling is a very satisfying way to super clean your mouth. The toxins and microbes dissolve in the oil as it is swished between the teeth. You spit this out, complete with murky debris, and then freshen the mouth. That's all there is to it!

What you need:

Coconut oil, bicarbonate of soda, toothbrush/toothpaste

How to do it:

Oil pulling can be done first thing in the morning, or last thing at night, on an empty stomach. Place 1 tbsp of coconut oil in the mouth and swish it between your teeth. (It quickly turns to a liquid.) Do not swallow, just work the oil around your mouth for 10 minutes. Then spit it out.

Dissolve 1 tsp of bicarbonate in a little warm water, swish this between your teeth then spit it out.

Clean your teeth thoroughly with a toothbrush and toothpaste and enjoy the feeling of a very clean mouth.

Note: I have recently switched to an Oral B electric toothbrush and personally find this to be more effective than a regular toothbrush.

5. Rebounding

We've already mentioned the benefits of exercise to health. Rebounding on a mini trampoline is a gentle exercise that can be done by just about everyone and it helps with posture, oxygenation and muscle strength. It is also particularly effective at stimulating lymphatic flow, which has very positive effects on detoxification.

Mini trampolines are widely available and take up very little floor space. Try building short spells into your day; maybe play some favourite music, or even rebound when watching the TV. What could be simpler?

6. Enemas

Enemas are not for everybody, and to some they may sound a bit weird. But for the serious detoxer who is actively seeking to move their health into a new dimension, enemas offer a simple and effective way to reduce your toxic load by stimulating liver function and cleansing the bowel.

Many naturopathic doctors report that once patients get over their initial reservations or inhibitions, enemas soon become one of their favourite parts of therapy. Detox fans report an emotional benefit from colon cleansing too, becoming more mentally alert and of clearer mind.

Enemas were part of mainstream medical practice until 1972, when laxative drugs took their place. Interestingly though, a recent study utilised coffee enema alongside medication in endoscopy. The coffee solution reaches the liver via the hepatic portal vein, resulting in dilatation of the bile ducts. It also stimulates gut motility and bile drainage. Those patients administered coffee enemas had significantly cleaner intestines, due to more efficient bile removal, versus those taking laxatives only.[96] This study supports the action of coffee on bile production and also comments on safety. Patients were assessed one week after receiving the enema and none of them experienced any adverse effects from the therapy.

When administered rectally, very little of the caffeine enters the blood stream, as it is metabolised quite differently to when taken as a beverage. A study comparing blood caffeine levels in healthy male subjects showed rectal infusion was 3.5 times lower than when consumed orally.[97]

Two important considerations when preparing enemas for home use are to cool the water to body temperature, and disinfect all equipment well to prevent risk of infection. It is best to do the enema after a bowel movement.

I now discuss how to go about doing a coffee enema. In the early stages you may prefer to start either with plain (bottled) water or chamomile tea (cooled to body temperature) for a gentler cleanse, and to get used to it.

Relax! You're in the privacy of your own bathroom and no-one can see you!

What you need:

Enema kit from Manifest Health (see resources), lubrication (eg: aloe jelly, olive oil), bottled water, organic coffee and probiotics.

How to do an enema:

1. Prepare a jug of filtered black coffee using 2 tablespoons of an organic blend and 600ml of bottled water. Allow it to cool to body temperature; adding some ice cubes can speed this up.

2. Choose a suitable space near the bathroom, with a door handle on which to hang the enema bag. Use towels, blankets and pillows to make it comfortable. Have a good book or music to listen to.

3. Pour the coffee solution into the enema bag and hang this on the door handle (tap closed).

4. Remove air bubbles from the tube by opening the tap and allowing liquid to run back into the jug. Once the bubbles have gone, close the tap and pour the coffee back into the enema bag.

5. Lie down on your left side in a foetal position. Lubricate your anus and the enema tip, then gently insert the tip 2- 4 inches.

6. Open the valve and allow the liquid to flow into the rectum.

7. Initially you may only be able to hold the solution for a few minutes, but, with practice, extend this up to 15- 20 minutes. You can read or listen to music to pass the time.

8. Then evacuate by going to the toilet. No need to hurry, again just relax and let things happen.

9. Disinfect the enema kit after use and drink plenty of water or herbal tea. It is good practice to take a probiotic to enhance your gut flora.

Enemas are widely used in naturopathic circles and are a key part of the Gerson therapy. I believe that they are very helpful when you are actively detoxing. This technique ensures that bile flow is optimised and waste products are excreted efficiently to prevent any recirculation, also known as auto-intoxication.

Enjoy!

Summary

This section should empower you to become involved in your own healthcare and make simple changes to help create an environment which is hostile to cancer. These include:

1. Boost your immune system with probiotics, Vitamin C, Vitamin D, medicinal mushrooms and plant-based antioxidants.

2. Follow an alkaline diet which is plant based with moderate amounts of high quality protein from plant and / or animal sources.

3. Cut out sugar! This doesn't mean that you are denied treats, just that you are more discerning about quality.

4. Eat a nutrient rich diet with plenty of fresh, whole foods to support liver health and detoxification.

5. Remember to breathe!

6. Consider some easy 'at-home' ways to boost your detoxification, from oil pulling to skin brushing and enemas.

Chapter Three:
Eat Real Food -
What We Need and Why

Over years of working in nutritional healthcare, I have often found myself encouraging people to 'eat like their grandparents did.'

Fifty years ago pretty much all the food we ate was natural. My Grandma always had a pot of soup on the stove (and Grandad made homemade toffee but at least it was made with butter and not processed or industrialised oils!) As a child in the 70s, we mostly ate real food, but I can remember processed foods creeping in; Mum and Dad enjoying a Vesta pack of Chinese noodles as a Saturday night treat, the advent of freezers, which meant food was more accessible, and boil in the bag fish in parsley sauce. For mash get Smash!

Today, many kids almost think that food grows in the supermarket! **The dominance of refined carbohydrates and low fat fayre is killing us.** The issues we face today are a slow, insidious compromise of health with far reaching consequences. And this is despite the incredible standard of living that we enjoy in the Western world.

So it's time to get real in the kitchen. The food manufacturers would have you believe that you don't have time to cook for yourself, and with both parents now working as the norm, it may feel like there is some truth in this. You just need to know how to throw good food together easily and fast. Your Granny didn't have a dishwasher, Magimix and slow cooker! But you can make use of time-saving modern gadgets. Bulk cook and freeze. Find a way that works for you.

Let's start with some real understanding of the healthy 'real food' way to eat, giving you some theory to underpin your meal planning. Much of this discussion is grounded in general health, but we will also consider some pertinent thoughts relating to cancer – animal versus vegetarian protein, whether or not you should eat dairy, the problem with grains, managing alcohol, and organic or not?

The Macronutrients: Fats, Carbs and Proteins

There are three main food groups, taught in every school in the land. Most diets are a play on these three variables – low fat, high protein, low carb etc. But the truth is you need a balance of all three, as they all perform different roles in your body.

Dietary Fat

For most of the last thirty or so years we have, been actively advised to eat low fat foods and, in particular, avoid saturated and animal fats in favour of polyunsaturated vegetable oils. The case against fat has been made by virtue of its name (assumed to make you fat), its calorie content and some persuasive public health messages originating in the 1950s.

On a per gram basis, fat contains more than double the calories of protein and carbohydrate:

> Fat – 9.5 calories
>
> Carbohydrate – 4.2 calories

Protein – 4.1 calories

Fat consumption became an ideal candidate for a target as obesity levels in the Western world rose. The assumption was that by cutting out fat we would lose any excess pounds. This is the 'calories in / calories out' theory.

At the same time, a compelling story was launched linking fat intake to heart disease. Ancel Keys was an American scientist who studied the influence of diet on health. He is most famous for *his Seven Countries* study, which appeared to show that a high level of serum cholesterol was strongly related to heart disease mortality.[98] It was hypothesized that high cholesterol levels resulted from a diet high in animal fats. The low fat mantra was thus established by the American Heart Association and then taken on board by governments around the world.

It is now increasingly becoming evident that this theory is completely incorrect and the consequences are evident in the increasing levels of obesity, diabetes and cancer we see today.

For a start, there were a total of twenty two countries for which data was gathered, but it appears that Keys cherry picked the countries which fitted his theory, whilst excluding those that actually showed an inverse relationship between fat intake and heart disease. When all twenty-two countries were included, the apparent link between fat and heart disease vanished.[99]

The calorie argument doesn't hold either. This supposes that by reducing calories, either by eating less or moving more, weight would be lost (or gained if calories were increased). In 1936 an experiment with fasting, obese mice was undertaken. Their food was dramatically restricted. The expectation was that they would simply be able to burn body fat to survive. Instead they died of starvation despite still being obese; clearly they were unable to access their own fat stores. [100]

Another study in the late 1960s overfed eight prison convicts with up to 10,000 calories a day. This is four times the calorie intake recommended for an average man. After 30 weeks, two had easily gained weight but six of the subjects had gained no more than a few pounds despite the significant overfeeding.[101] This demonstrated that there is more to weight loss, or gain, than the calorie content of the food eaten. Metabolism affects how much of a nutrient is either burned for fuel, or stored as fat. Hence, penalising fat for having higher calories per gram just doesn't make any sense.

It is interesting to consider how public health advice could have been so catastrophically incorrect. Denise Minger, in her book *'Death by Food Pyramid: How Shoddy Science, Sketchy Politics & Shady Special Interests Ruined Your Health'*[102], has researched this thoroughly and explains the whole pathway by which the advice was developed. Tom Naughton, entertainer turned health educator, in his talk *'Diet, Health & the Wisdom of* Crowds', gives a brilliant (and entertaining) insight into why people are turning away from established health advice.[103]

Good vs Bad Fats

We'll go on to look at the roles fat performs in your body, but before then, let's take a moment to consider whether or not all fats are equal.

Firstly, what is a fat? Fats and oils are long chains of atoms including carbon, hydrogen and oxygen. The universal characteristic of all fat is simply that they are foods or food components that are 'fatty' or 'oily'. As such they don't dissolve in or mix with water.

Saturated fats are strong and rigid because they are 'saturated' with the maximum number of hydrogen atoms. This makes them very stable and safe to heat. They are usually the storage medium of an animal (an exception is coconut oil).

Unsaturated fats include double bond(s) within their structure, where hydrogen atoms are missing. This makes their molecules more flexible, hence they are liquid at room temperature. They are more prone to rancidity than animal fats, and can be oxidised when heated. Olive oil is a monounsaturated oil (one point of unsaturation) and can be heated gently. Vegetable oils, like sunflower oil or rapeseed oil, are polyunsaturated oils (multiple points of unsaturation), and hence highly unstable at temperature. Heating is not recommended, as these oils become oxidised and produce toxic compounds, which are detrimental to health.[104] Some of the compounds produced, such as malondialdehyde, are carcinogenic.

Margarines are made from vegetable oils (liquid at room temperature), which are chemically processed into a solid form (to give a butter like consistency). We are now seeing a complete reversal on the advice to eat margarine, with TIME magazine running the headline 'Butter is Back'.[105] This is because butter is not only a more natural product, but it is better for health too.[106]

The essential fats – omega 3 and omega 6 - are polyunsaturates, which are vital for good health but cannot be made in the body (hence it is essential that they are eaten). Omega 3 oils are found predominantly in fish, flax seeds, pumpkin seeds and walnuts. Omega 6 oils are found in nuts, seeds, eggs and meat. To protect the oils in nuts and seeds from oxidation consider keeping them in glass jars in the fridge. It is fine to use them in whole form in cooking (such as baking), but do not heat seed or nut oils (which would then be oxidised). Flax oil should always be refrigerated, or better still kept in the freezer. If you use ground nuts or seeds keep them refrigerated too, and if possible grind just small batches as and when you need them. Always buy fish oils from a reputable source to ensure that they have been efficiently stabilised. Some fish oils may need refrigerating.

In essence, 'good' fats are natural – including those from fish, animals, nuts, seeds, avocados and olive or coconut oil. 'Bad' fats are either oils that have been heated to high temperatures or have undergone chemical processing such as hydrogenation. You might like to look on the label for 'cold pressed' or 'extracted by mechanical means' when selecting oils, which means that they haven't been subjected to such processes.

Benefits of Fats and Oils

1. Good quality fat helps you to feel full up, which is a useful way to curb excessive eating. With fat in your meals you feel more satisfied for longer, and are less likely to suffer from food cravings, which tend to be exacerbated by high carbohydrate diets.

2. Every cell in your body is contained within a membrane which is made up of the essential fatty acids. The membrane plays an important role in controlling the molecules that can enter and leave the cell. It needs to have the right balance of fats to retain flexibility.

3. Up to 60% of your brain is made of fat.[107] Some studies show that cholesterol, particularly HDL, is important in enhancing cognition and memory.[108]

4. Many key hormones in your body are derived from cholesterol. These include the stress hormone cortisol, and all of your sex hormones.

5. Some fat helps to protect organs and is a reserve for energy. Fatty acids can be broken down to provide fuel by a process called beta-oxidation. This enables you to go for periods without eating, without loss of performance.

6. Fat soluble vitamins can, by definition, only be absorbed when you eat fat. You can become deficient in Vitamins A, D and E when you eat a low fat diet, even if these vitamins are present in the food you ingest.

Does Fat Consumption Increase Inflammation?

Omega 3 and 6 fatty acids are the precursors of prostaglandins – hormone like molecules which are either anti- or pro-inflammatory, so together they manage inflammation in the body. Omega 3 oils including fish oils are renowned for their anti-inflammatory action, whereas arachidonic acid, an omega 6 fat derived from animal products, can be pro-inflammatory. It's all about getting a balance and, where possible, selecting meat which has been predominantly grass fed (corn feeding will increase levels of omega 6).

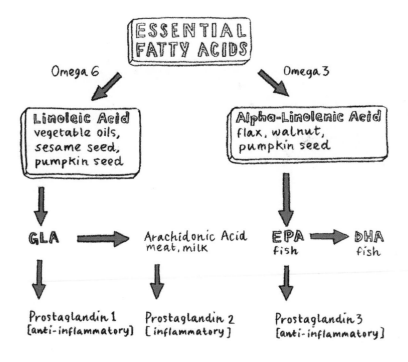

Fig 4: Essential fatty acid pathways

Dietary Carbohydrate

Carbohydrate is currently the dominant food in our diet and the one that we are most encouraged to eat.

It comprises complex carbohydrates such as starch (found in vegetables, cereals, bread and pasta) and simple carbohydrates, such as sugar (found in sweet foods).

The carbohydrate element of any food is broken down by digestion into its smallest unit of glucose or sugar, and is transported around the body in the blood stream (hence blood glucose or blood sugar). The main role of carbohydrate, and why it is so significant, is to produce energy. It is your primary source of fuel, but not the only one. More about this in Chapter Seven.

Interestingly, there is only the equivalent of 2 teaspoons of sugar or glucose in your blood at any one time. This is why there is so much concern about the amount of sugar being eaten in the average diet. Five grams of carbohydrate roughly equates to a teaspoon of sugar, and this can be a handy way to assess a food's sugar impact. Recently there has been considerable media coverage about the hidden sugars in our foods, and this includes savoury as well as sweet foods. A survey of supermarket ready meals showed that some contain up to 10 tsp of sugar, which is more than a bar of Dairy Milk or a can of Cola.[109]

Excessive sugar intake wreaks havoc with your glucose metabolism, and is believed to be the main culprit that is driving diabetes, obesity and chronic ill health. As we've already discussed, sugar feeds cancer cells, hence watching carbohydrate intake is an essential component of the *Outsmart Cancer* strategy.

Low GL

As I mentioned in Chapter Two, a low Glycaemic Load (GL) diet is favourable for good health. It should focus on carbohydrates from plant based sources and may include some fruit and grains (more on this later). All fruit and vegetables contain carbs, and starchy veg, such as sweet potato, squash and carrots, are concentrated sources.

In addition to minimising swings in blood sugar levels, fruits and vegetables are packed full of vitamins and minerals, the very nutrients your body needs in abundance to work efficiently and effectively.

What About Fibre?

Fibre is the indigestible part of a carbohydrate, and serves a role in promoting bowel health. There are two types of fibre – soluble and insoluble.

Soluble fibre attracts water and forms a gel, which tends to slow the movement through the digestive system. It is readily fermented in the colon or large intestine by your bowel bacteria. It helps with the excretion of cholesterol, bile acids and products of detoxification, such as hormones, by binding with them and preventing their reabsorption into the blood stream. Once fermented, short chain fatty acids (SCFA) are produced, which play numerous roles in health including:

• Stabilising glucose levels
• Nourishing the intestinal cells and improving the barrier properties of the colonic mucosal layer (protecting against 'leaky gut')
• Stimulating immune cells
• Suppressing cholesterol synthesis

Food sources include oats, lentils, berries, apples, pears, psyllium, cucumber, celery and carrots.

Insoluble fibre passes through the digestive tract relatively unchanged, adding bulk to the stool and speeding up transit time. This is helpful for relieving constipation. Food sources include whole grains, bran, couscous, brown rice, bulgur, courgette, celery, broccoli, cabbage, onions, tomato, green leafy vegetables and fruit.

Net Carbs

A useful way of assessing the sugar impact of a food is to consider net carbs, defined by the late Mr Atkins[110] as total carbs less the fibre. It's not the whole story, as the speed of sugar release, known as the Glycaemic Index (or GI) is also important. But, as GI values are not stated on food labels, this measure is a useful 'rough and ready' indicator.

For example, consider a granola bar where:

> Total carbs = 26g
>
> Fibre = 3g
>
> Net carbs = 23g (26g- 3g)

With an average teaspoon of sugar weighing 5g, this equates to roughly 4.5 tsps of sugar per bar. Always aim to keep sugar intake low, and offset its impact by choosing foods with protein and fat content too, which slows down the sugar release.

Dietary Protein

The third of the macronutrients is protein. This word comes from the Greek 'proteos', meaning 'of prime importance', and it is truly an important building block in the human body. Good sources of protein include meat, fish, nuts, seeds, dairy, eggs and pulses or beans.

When we eat these foods, our digestion breaks them down into amino acids, which are then absorbed through the digestive tract. These amino acids perform a whole host of functions to keep us fit and well, from growth and repair, to learning and memory, to replicating our DNA and more.

An analogy would be taking a model house made out of Lego, breaking it down into Lego bricks, and then making a new model of a plane or car. In the same way, when we eat protein, say in the form of cheese or eggs, we break the proteins down into amino acids and rebuild them into hair, skin and nails. How very clever!

All animal and plant life is constructed from a total of 21 amino acids which are grouped into essential, conditionally-essential, and non-essential categories. The 8 essential amino acids are exactly that – they cannot be made, and so must be obtained from the diet. Those that are conditionally-essential are not normally required in the diet but may be required under certain conditions – such as infant prematurity or for an individual in severe catabolic stress, where muscle mass in being broken down to fuel energy requirements in the body.

What Does Protein Do?

1. **Structure:** Just as a house is made of bricks, you are made of amino acids, which give you structure and form. The obvious place for protein is in your muscle mass, but even bone and joint health requires a source of amino acids.

2. **Enzymes:** These are responsible for thousands of metabolic processes that sustain life. They act as catalysts to speed up chemical reactions in your body, from digesting your food to synthesising DNA. Most of them are made from protein.

3. **Hormones:** Protein based hormones include insulin to manage your blood glucose levels, thyroxine to control your metabolic rate and the stress hormone adrenaline.

4. **Neurotransmitters:** These are molecules which transmit signals between brain cells and so are responsible for mood, memory and thinking ability. Not all neurotransmitters are protein based, but some of the important ones are, including

serotonin (the happy hormone) and dopamine (reward and motivation).

5. A natural way to support mood is to ensure regular protein intake, together with vitamins and minerals, which support the conversion of amino acids into neurotransmitters. This is why mood and feelings of wellbeing usually dramatically improve on a real food diet containing macronutrients and plentiful vitamins and minerals.

6. ***Immunity:*** Protein based anti-bodies keep your immune system functioning well.

Having established the macronutrients required within an *Outsmart Cancer* diet, we are now going to explore some of the controversies which abound in the media. By presenting you with more background on each of these issues, you are free to make decisions which are right for you.

Controversy 1: Protein – Animal or Vegetable?

There is much debate about whether an animal protein or vegetarian diet is healthier.

A low fat, plant based diet has, in the past, been a dominant model of therapeutic eating, and this is how I was initially trained. But new research is starting to throw up very interesting results based on meat eating, higher fat and even ketogenic diets. Ketogenic refers to the use of fat as a primary fuel and the resulting production of ketone bodies.

Personally I enjoy both vegetarian and animal sources of protein, alongside lots of vegetables, and it is interesting to consider the merits of each.

Whole Food, Plant Based Diets

Two significant opinion formers in promoting a meat free diet are Dean Ornish MD and Colin Campbell PhD. Dean Ornish is an American physician well known for his lifestyle approach to controlling coronary heart disease. Published in The Lancet in 1990, his clinical research provided some of the first evidence that changes in diet and lifestyle have a significant impact on health. His methods include a whole food, plant based diet, smoking cessation, moderate exercise, plus psychological and emotional stress management support, including yoga and meditation. Not only did participants enjoy a reduced level of cardiac events, but there were also clinical signs of the reversal of heart disease with reduced atherosclerosis (narrowing of the arteries) after one year. In contrast, the control group saw progression of their disease.[111]

In 2005, Ornish went on to show the impact of diet and lifestyle changes for prostate cancer, again utilising a whole food, plant based diet. A total of 93 volunteers were recruited with early, low grade prostate cancer and assigned either to an experimental group with extensive diet & lifestyle support, or to a group given standard advice by their physician.

This study showed a dramatically positive result from lifestyle intervention, and I mentioned this when exploring why nutrition is important, in Chapter One. The advice and support received by the experimental group included:

- Vegan diet with protein powder

- Supplements – *fish oil 3g, vit E, selenium, vit C*

- Moderate exercise – *walking 30 mins, 6 days per week*

- Stress management – *60 mins daily*

- Weekly support group

The control group had none of this intervention. Clearly there are many differences between the two groups, and it cannot be known whether there would be any impact – positive or negative – from including a moderate amount of animal protein alongside all of this support.

T. Colin Campbell is an American biochemist and author of *The China Study*. He was brought up as a meat eater on a dairy farm and transitioned to a vegan diet during his adult life. His nutritional philosophy is based around whole, plant based foods.

Campbell's early work was based on animal models. In one study, rats were dosed with the cancer promoter aflatoxin, and fed either a low or high casein (milk protein) diet. Over a 100 week study period (the average lifespan of a rat) those fed 5% protein were alive and active whilst all those fed 20% protein were either dead or near death. Those switched from high-protein to low-protein at either 40 or 60 weeks had 35-40% less tumour growth than those fed high-protein only.[112] This study raises potential concerns over dairy and cancer, but cannot be extrapolated to caution against all animal products in humans.

The China Study was Campbell's greatest work; an epidemiological study with questionnaires, blood tests and urine samples taken from 6,500 adults. These included direct measurement of food intake over a three-day period.[113]

The China Study provides a unique opportunity to investigate associations between dietary habits and disease (this is not the same as causation – just because two attributes are associated, does not mean that one necessarily causes the other). The book, though, is a bit confusing, as it draws from many sources, not just the China Study, and supports the viewpoint that a plant based diet is associated with greater health benefits. Most often comparisons are made between diets in China versus America, rather than an insightful study of the extensive Chinese data. I was left with the overall sense that this book is less about a comparison of a low versus a high protein diet, but instead between whole foods (China) and a diet with a very high proportion of junk food and poor dietary habits (US).

It's worth noting that there has been criticism of Campbell's interpretation of the China Study data. Denise Minger has accessed the raw data from Oxford and undertaken her own analysis. She doesn't have the same academic standing as Campbell, but her views, published as a blog post, are interesting all the same. In this analysis, a positive number is associated with cancer risk, with a higher number indicating higher risk.

For example, considering lifestyle factors that are associated with breast cancer, Minger notes that the China study showed a correlation with dietary fat at +18 and with animal protein at +12, which are not statistically significant. But there are several other variables which are more positively associated with breast cancer risk, and yet these factors are ignored in Campbell's review:

Blood glucose level +36

Alcohol intake +31

Yearly fruit consumption +25

Processed starch and sugar intake +20

Dietary fat intake +18

Legume intake +17

Animal protein intake +12

The higher positive number is more strongly associated with breast cancer risk.[114]

This exposes a potential for researcher bias, where results may be selected based on an already established position.

And finally, it's worth mentioning that many studies into vegetarian diets examine the health of Seventh Day Adventists. One such study showed results in favour of a vegetarian diet, but found that this group ate more wholefoods and had a lower intake of processed foods, including doughnuts. Again such confounding factors can potentially skew results, and the study acknowledges that better health in the vegetarian group cannot be ascribed only to the absence of meat.[115]

Whole Food, Plant Based Diets with Animal Protein

In 2012, Dr Terry Wahls hit You Tube with her Ted talk – Minding your Mitochondria. Her 17 minute story of how she used food to recover from secondary progressive Multiple Sclerosis has seen, to date, nearly 2 million views.[116]

Dr Wahls is a clinical professor at the University of Iowa and was diagnosed with relapsing remitting MS in 2000. Despite the very best medical interventions, including chemotherapy in an attempt to slow the disease, her illness progressed, unrelentingly. She began using a tilt recline wheelchair because of weakness in her back muscles, and it was clear that she was heading to becoming bedridden.

After exhausting the medical literature in search of a way to arrest her descent, Dr Wahls turned to nutritional research and added vitamins and minerals to her schedule, which slowed the decline. In 2007 she discovered functional medicine, which seeks to establish the root cause of illness and address nutritional imbalances, and she redesigned her diet along paleo lines. Paleo is a far cry from today's modern diet and goes back to a time of natural foods – the caveman diet. It excludes all grains, dairy, processed foods and sugars and instead focuses on pasture raised meat, fish, vegetables (lots of them), fruits, particularly berries, nuts and seeds. Fat, including saturated animal fat, is positively encouraged.

Dr Wahls' recovery was nothing short of remarkable. Within a year she was able to walk without a cane and even completed an 18 mile bike ride. Today she is fit and well, and her work now focuses on running clinical trials to assess the impact of diet on disease.

Wahls' story is a powerful message that what you eat can either promote or rob you of good health, and the solution that worked for her flies in the face of current dietary advice. Her disease was directly caused by a lack of vital nutrients including animal proteins and fats, which enable her body, and her mitochondria (the organelles in your cells which make energy) to function optimally.

She is not the only one. The internet is teaming with stories of people who have exhausted medical resources and brought about their own healing through nutrition, including eating animal protein. Examples include Dr Mark Hyman (chronic fatigue)[117], Danielle Walker (ulcerative colitis)[118] and Sarah Ballantyne PhD (autoimmune disease).[119] I consistently see this in my clinic, where moving to a plant based diet with moderate animal protein results in significant health improvements.

But - What About Cancer?

We often hear screaming headlines about meat, particularly red meat, and health issues including cancer. But just consider, prior to Terry Wahls' experience, the main dietary recommendation for MS was low in fat, with restricted meat, and plentiful whole grains[120] - the polar opposite of her experience. Could such a paradox also be confusing the picture with cancer? I think it can.

For instance, the *Nurse's Health Study* investigated 88,803 premenopausal women and found an association between meat consumption and breast cancer.[121] As I said earlier, just because two things are linked through association, doesn't mean that one necessarily causes the other. One of the biggest issues with this kind of study is that it doesn't consider other foods within the diet, and this might have a significant influence. In Chapter Three, I proposed that red meat consumption is often a burger served with highly inflammatory and acidic foods –a white bun, chips, soda. So this, if true, would most definitely skew the results in respect of cancer risk, just like it did in the Seventh Day Adventist study mentioned earlier.

We are currently lacking well designed cancer trials to truly evaluate a real food, plant based diet including animal protein. Based on what I see in practice every day, I cannot demonise well husbanded and unprocessed animal protein, provided it is within the context of a high plant intake. As we'll see later, meat is one of the most nutritious foods on the planet! The World Cancer Research Fund advises up to 300g of red meat per person per week, which equates to 2-3 portions.[122] So if you enjoy meat, feel comfortable to include it in moderation within your diet, alongside other proteins for variety.

On the other hand if you prefer a vegetarian diet, that's fine too, but be particularly careful to obtain adequate sources of dietary protein. Extreme protein deficiency can have dire consequences, and hence I'm sharing this experience from an ex-vegan.

Potential Negative Consequences of a Long Term Vegan Diet

Ex-vegan, Lierre Keith, wrote her book, *The Vegetarian Myth*[123], in part as a cautionary tale. The negative consequences of her dietary choices were degenerative joint disease, hypoglycaemia (low blood sugar), hormonal problems (she stopped menstruating three months into a vegan diet), itchy skin, digestive problems, anxiety and depression. She has recovered in part by returning to a nutrient dense paleo style diet, but some of the damage is lifelong.

Keith's book is more than just her story. She also goes into the consequences of current agricultural methods. Whilst many may adopt a vegetarian diet to avoid animal cruelty, she urges people to look at the bigger picture. The dominance of mono crops in agriculture – corn, soy and the like, has decimated the agricultural landscape and with it the erosion of wildlife, birds, bugs and worms which play a vital part in our ecosystem. Instead, she argues, we should demand high standards for animal husbandry, and accept that we are part of that very same ecosystem. Plants turn the energy of the sun into food. Herbivores become food for omnivores/ carnivores. Living matter becomes nutrients for the soil. Ashes to ashes. Dust to dust.

Controversy 2: Should You Eat Dairy?

When I was diagnosed with cancer in 2003, I came across a book called *'Your Life in Your Hands'* by Jane Plant.[124] This highlighted Jane's own success with a no-dairy diet in the remission of her cancer. She reasoned that Chinese populations had a very low rate of breast cancer compared to the West, and theorised that their lack of dairy was a potential cause of this. She reports that within 6 weeks of her new diet the lump in her neck had receded and she was cancer free within a year.

Jane's experience is enormously inspiring, and whilst it is great that this worked for her, is it right to write off dairy completely, all of the time?

I initially followed Jane's advice, and I'm glad that I did, but I have a broader view now too.

Digestion and Intolerance

A key indicator that you should try going dairy free is if you have underlying health issues such as asthma or skin problems, digestive issues such as bloating, constipation or diarrhoea, or excessive mucus. These issues often relate back to gut health, and whether you have a foul bowel or a well-functioning system. An overgrowth of unfriendly bacteria will mean that lactose, the sugar in dairy, ferments in the digestive tract, causing problems.

This may be caused by a lack of digestive efficiency, gut dysbiosis (disruption of the normal bowel flora), or a deficiency of the enzyme lactase (a genetic consequence).

People with a family history of coeliac disease may also need to be cautious, as milk can be cross reactive with gluten. The milk protein casein is similar in structure to gluten and can invoke an immune response similar to gluten exposure. Around 50% of coeliac patients are also sensitive to dairy.[125]

Whilst it is important to resolve digestive issues (unless arising genetically), milk products can be made more digestible by fermentation. This involves the action of good bacteria on lactose, the milk sugar and was historically used as a preservation method. We are all familiar with yoghurt which contains probiotics. Kefir is another probiotic milk drink with amazing health benefits. In addition to good bacteria, it is rich in vitamins, minerals and amino acids. (More about this in Chapter Six).

Hormones

There is concern about the oestrogenic activity of dairy products, particularly of cow's milk. Indeed when cow's milk was introduced to prostate cancer cells in vitro, a 30% increase in tumour cell proliferation was noted. This was also the case for soya. However, almond milk exposure resulted in a 30% decrease in cell activity.[126] Fortunately, there is now a wide range of nut milks available on the market, and they are also very easy, and quite delicious, to make at home.

Goat and sheep products can also be a good choice from a health point of view. In a study comparing different milks, goat was found to be significantly less oestrogenic, with the authors concluding *"Goat milk represents a better dietary choice for individuals concerned with limiting their oestrogen intake."*[127]

Goat's milk is generally regarded as easier to digest than cows and many practitioners report this to be the case in clinical practice. Reasons for this may be the lack of a protein, alpha S1 casein, in goat's (and human) milk, or the smaller fat globules in goat's milk.[128]

Nutritional Value

From a nutritional point of view, dairy is an excellent source of protein, which is one of the key reasons I advocate some goats and sheep's products like cheese or yoghurt, provided they are well tolerated. It can be a convenient contribution to a fast meal, and many people really enjoy the creamy texture and taste. **Think Roquefort melted over pears and mixed into a salad, or a goat's cheese spread on crackers and topped with mango.**

Dairy is also prized for its calcium content, but I find this to be less compelling, as there are many alternative calcium sources, and these foods often also have a superior magnesium level too:

Minerals per 100g dry weight:

	Calcium (mg)	Magnesium (mg)
Cow's milk	1,105	105
Sesame seed	702	388
Okra	1,194	530
Curly kale	1,121	293
Spinach	1,651	524
Mustard & Cress	1,064	468
Watercress	2,266	200

Source: The composition of food. FSA. (3rd edition)

So, in a nutshell, consider significantly reducing or eliminating cow's dairy from your diet, unless you are using it in fermented products such as yoghurt or kefir and then only choose organic. There are now plenty of non-dairy milk alternatives readily available in the supermarket, from coconut to almond and hazelnut. Coconut cream is great for a more creamy texture. You may also like to include moderate amounts of goat's and sheep's cheese and yoghurt, unless you find that these products don't agree with you, in which case they can be avoided.

Controversy 3: Aren't Grains Good for You?

Healthy eating guidelines currently encourage you to eat "plenty of starchy foods such as bread, rice, potato and pasta."[129]

This advice was based on the Food Guide Pyramid of 1992, which was developed not by Public Health departments, but by the US Department of Agriculture (USDA). Six to eleven portions of starchy carbohydrates were recommended on a daily basis, which basically nets down to continuous carb loading through meals and snacks. I think that this nutritional advice is responsible for increasing levels of blood sugar chaos, obesity, diabetes and ill health; exactly the health problems that are currently seen on a grand scale.

In the UK, the NHS now promote the Eatwell plate, but grains still have a prominent position occupying one third of the plate. Such guidelines promote the notion that grains are good for you, when in fact, for many of us, this is just not the case.

Depending on your current state of health, activity levels and genetic disposition, a high grain based diet may have undesirable health consequences for the following reasons:

1. High carb = sugar

Grains are very dense carbohydrates, and this food group comprises an average of 85% of their dry weight:

	% carbohydrate
Wheat	74%
Rice (brown)	94%
Rye	89%
Oats	72%

Hence eating grains will always mean you run the risk of having disrupted blood sugar levels, causing big swings in glucose levels especially when they are eaten in typical UK sized portions. The more complex the grain, the slower the sugar release, as it takes longer for your digestion to break the food down. Hence, rye bread is a better choice than wheat, and oats a better choice than cereals. But even then, I recommend controlling portion sizes.

Most people don't associate a piece of bread with sugar. David Perlmetter MD, author of Grain Brain[130], highlights this when giving lectures to the medical profession. He shows a slide with photos of four common foods – a slice of whole bread, a snickers bar, a tablespoon of sugar and a banana and asks the audience to guess which food gives the biggest surge in blood sugar. They are surprised to learn that it is bread, with a Glycaemic Index of 71, which trumps the pack!

2. Low in Micronutrients

Compared to vegetables, grains are an inferior source of many micronutrients and this is the reason that bread and cereals are often fortified with vitamins. For example, wheat contains no retinol, the precursor of vitamin A, less than half of the vitamin B6 of carrots and a mere 17% of the vitamin E of broccoli.

Vitamin	Wheat	Carrot	Broccoli
Retinol (vit A)	0	79559	4873
E	1.88	5.49	11.02
B1	.55	.98	.85
B2	.1	.1	.51
B3	6.63	1.96	7.63
B6	.58	1.37	1.18
Folate	66.3	117.6	762.8
B5	.93	2.45	0
Biotin	8.14	5.88	0
C	0	58.8	737.3

Source: The composition of food. FSA. (3rd edition)

3. Grains are Dominant

Consider a tuna and tomato sandwich compared to a tuna salad. The dominant food in the sandwich is the bread, which crowds out other more health giving foods by filling you up (at least in the short term). Your sandwich may have all the goodness of a half a tomato at most. In contrast, a salad is full of vegetables which are all teaming with micro nutrients to help your body work efficiently and effectively.

4. Grains Potentially Promote Inflammation

Grain intolerance, particularly to wheat, is a significant issue to many and can be an underlying cause of digestive issues, obesity and ill health.

William Davis MD has written extensively on this topic.[131] His book *Wheat Belly* talks about the issues with the development of the wheat grain in production today. This has been hybridised to increase yields but also, he believes, now has a significant allergenic potential for many people.

In susceptible people, wheat and other grains may contribute to the manifestation of chronic inflammation by increasing intestinal permeability and initiating a pro-inflammatory immune response.[132]

We all have a different tolerance for grains. Young, lean and fit individuals may do well with more grain in their diet. Regular exercise increases insulin sensitivity and this could help to negate some of their glycaemic effect in people with a strong metabolism. But others do better on a low or no grain regime. This need not compromise fibre levels (an objection often mooted to low grain diets) provided vegetable intake is high.

Before I was diagnosed with cancer, sandwiches were a staple lunch for me, but now that would be quite unusual.

Fear not, there are much better lunches than sandwiches! If you are striving for wheat or gluten free, then nut or seed flours can make delicious alternatives to bread or crackers. One of our favourite lunches at the *Outsmart Cancer* workshop consists of wraps made with gram flour, gluten free and derived from chick peas (recipes in Chapter Five and online).

Controversy 4: Alcohol

Many of us enjoy an alcoholic beverage, and drinking has been a pastime within human civilisation for millennia. For some it helps to ease social situations, or enables them to relax after a hard day's work. It creates bonds and a shared experience. It tastes quite nice too, and we enjoy it!

There is a general feeling that modest alcohol intake, particularly of red wine, may even be beneficial for health. However, the most recent study published in the British Medical Journal concludes that, with the exception of women over 65 drinking less than 10 units per week, there are no protective effects of alcohol. The authors explain that the industry norm is to include former drinkers and never drinkers as one homogenous group, whereas in reality reformed drinkers tend to have higher health risks. This has the result of overstating beneficial effects associated with a low consumption of alcohol.[133]

The potential ill effects of over consuming alcohol are well known, which is why Government advice encourages us to keep within limits. If you are healthy, then moderate drinking may work for you. This may be considerably less than you might think – it is the equivalent of a pint of beer (for a man) or one small glass of wine per day. Binge drinking (which has definite health consequences) is defined as 3 pints of beer, or 2 glasses of wine in one sitting.

But what does the available evidence linking cancer risk and alcohol tell us? Consider the findings of a 2012 meta-analysis of breast cancer risk and alcohol consumption. At just one glass a day, the risk was increased by 4%. However, at three glasses per day, the breast cancer risk increase is of the order of 40-50%. This translates into 5% or 50,000 cases of alcohol attributable cases worldwide.[134]

How to calculate units:

To work out the number of units of alcohol in a drink you will need to know both the volume and alcohol % (which is printed on the bottle or can). The number of units is the same as the alcohol % per litre, so simply scale down according to the drink volume ie: multiply the alcohol % by the drink volume (in ml), and divide by 1000 (or 1 litre):

250ml glass of wine (12%) = 3 units (12 x 250/1000)

568ml pint of beer (5%) = 2.8 units (5 x 568/1000)

Government guidelines are to keep weekly alcohol intake to below 14 units for a woman, and 21 units for a man. There are a number of apps which enable you to track your alcohol intake and help you to drink responsibly. The NHS Choices drinks tracker is a good one.

Alcohol and Cancer

I strongly advocate that if you have active cancer and are currently going through treatment, then you are well advised not to drink any alcohol at all. This may sound harsh, but just consider the following:

- Alcohol is classified by the International Agency for Research into Cancer (IARC) as a Group 1 carcinogen – which means that there is convincing evidence that it causes cancer in humans. Why would you want to expose yourself to more carcinogens when cancer is exactly what you are trying to recover from?

- It is a toxin which has to be detoxified in your liver to safely break it down and remove it from the body. This uses huge amounts of nutrients, including B vitamins and magnesium, which could be better deployed in helping to improve your health.

- It increases oestrogen levels, and promotes oxidative stress.[135]

- It provides empty calories – Drink Aware estimate a large glass of wine contains as many calories as a Cornetto ice cream. It also stimulates the appetite and may encourage over eating and hence weight gain.

- It is irritating to your gut, which may also be delicate during or following treatment.[136]

So, if you are in good health, then the odd social alcoholic drink is fine, provided your diet is good. But if you are working to improve your health then, with the exception of a very special occasion, alcohol is best avoided.

Controversy 5: Organic or Not?

The routine use of pesticides and herbicides in conventional agriculture has expanded to the extent that close to a billion pounds of toxic chemicals are introduced into the environment and our food supply every year.[137]

In contrast, organic foods are produced without the use of synthetic pesticides and chemical fertilisers, although the limited use of organically approved pesticides may be allowed. Organic produce also generally avoids processing using irradiation, industrial solvents or additives.

Does this 'cleaner' production process lead to 'cleaner' foods, which are less contaminated by chemicals and heavy metals? A recent meta-analysis of 343 peer-reviewed papers found this to be the case, and reported that non-organic produce carried *four times the pesticide levels* of its organic brethren.[138]

The same study also showed that organic produce carried lower levels of cadmium (a toxic heavy metal) and had a better nutrient profile, in particular with significantly higher levels of antioxidants.

Industrial chemicals are a driver of carcinogenesis (as highlighted in the WCRF report discussed in Chapter One), and so going organic is one way to reduce your own toxic exposure.

National organic box schemes are provided by Abel & Cole and Riverford, which deliver freshly farmed organic produce to your front door. Most of the major supermarkets now have a range of organic lines, and you may also have farms local to you.

The European Working Group (EWG) publishes an annual Shoppers Guide based on US Government data and lists the dirtiest, or most pesticide contaminated, fruits and vegetables.[139] In the 2015 review, nearly two thirds of the produce samples tested contained toxic residues, and 265 different chemicals were found.

This data is published as an easy to read 'Clean fifteen' and 'Dirty Dozen' list and it helps consumers to be able to make better choices when it comes to prioritising organic produce. For instance, avocados top the 'clean' list whilst apples are high up the 'dirty'. Full information can be found at www.ewg.org.

A further point worth mentioning here is that, if you are so inclined, 'grow your own' could be a good option. This could range from a few herbs on a windowsill, to turning over a small part of your garden, to renting an allotment.

Summary

This Chapter should build on your awareness of dietary factors. In it I have discussed issues pertinent both to general good health and to outsmarting cancer:

1. Dietary fat is essential for good health. It makes hormones, is a major component of brains and cell membranes, and helps you to absorb fat soluble vitamins.

2. Choose low glycaemic carbohydrates for fuel and fibre. Include lots of veg and some fruit to increase micronutrients and reduce or eliminate processed carbs.

3. You are made of protein – it builds structures, enzymes, neurotransmitters, antibodies and hormones.

4. Current research favours a plant based diet, but there is a growing awareness that some people do very well on a diet that also includes some animal protein. Go with what feels

right for you, but above all make sure your protein intake is sufficient.

5. It is good advice to restrict dairy products if you have digestive issues or active cancer. If you are healthy, then dairy is an excellent protein source and you may find goat or sheep products to be beneficial.

6. Wheat is probably an overrated product for most of us; it can limit overall nutrient intake and contribute to inflammation. Have it occasionally if you are healthy, but consider alternatives if your health is compromised.

7. Keep within Government guidelines for alcohol consumption, per week that is 21 units for a man and 14 units for a woman. Consider complete abstinence, save for a very special occasion, if your health is challenged.

8. Where possible shop organic and use the EWG guidelines to prioritise your choices. Don't stress if your budget doesn't stretch to organic or if organic supplies are not available. Just do your best and clean produce well before eating.

So now that you have some guidelines in place, we need to get more specific. The next section will clarify the wealth of fabulous foods that are available to you on the *Outsmart Cancer* eating plan. This will include a shopping guide, and recipes are available in Chapter Five. Also look for free bonus material online, including variations of the eating plan and more recipes.

Chapter Four:
The *Outsmart Cancer* Eating Plan

We're now at a stage in this book where I will help you to structure an eating plan, not a diet. This isn't about deprivation, it's about abundance! You'll be focussing on real food which is teaming with nutrients and delicious too. It can work well within a family setting, maybe with a little adjustment for others, if your little ones or partner are resistant to change.

As you transition you may need a little extra time to plan. Preparation can also be a consideration. Don't let this put you off – it's why every good kitchen has a selection of time saving gadgets. With a little practice you will become proficient at knocking meals together fast, and recipes are provided in Chapter Five to get you started.

By the end of this chapter you will have some eating guidelines and a shopping list. The list can be printed off online (see www.OutsmartCancer.co.uk) where I've also included variations such as vegetarian (excluding meat) and Paleo (excluding grains and dairy) diets.

This style of eating is how I eat most of the time (I'm sipping some chicken broth before lunch as I write this) and I've coached hundreds of clients on these principles too. Generally people report back that they feel satisfied more quickly, really enjoy the variety and quickly experience health benefits. These can include greater energy, improved digestion, better sleep and more balanced mood, for instance. All of these are important parameters in your journey towards optimum good health.

One question you might be thinking now is, am I allowed any treats? You most certainly are, but try to be discerning over quality. Good quality dark chocolate is, in moderation, a healthy choice, full of antioxidants, but if you really crave something that you know is not particularly good for you, then just have it occasionally (high days and holidays). If you find that this triggers an eating binge, then you may benefit from considering some emotional support, either from a friend, or professionally by working with a Nutritionist. There are lots of good quality treats you can make at home, where you can have confidence in the quality of the ingredients. One company worth checking out is UGG foods, who make the most wonderful cake and bread mixes using chia, almond and flax seeds (www.UggFoods.com, see Resources).

One thing I must stress, though, is that you don't beat yourself up if you make some bad food decisions. Just reflect on your actions and consider how you might make better choices next time.

The *Outsmart Cancer* Principles

1. Eat three good quality main meals a day, with an afternoon snack if required, all using unprocessed ingredients.

There may be situations when it is appropriate for you to eat little and often, particularly if you are going through treatment and not very hungry, or are struggling to maintain your weight. But for the most of us, we really do need to eat less often and in my experience eating three good meals a day (just like Granny did) is a fantastic way to optimise your health. If you are eating properly, you should easily be able to go 5 or 6 hours without thinking much about food. This is good feedback on whether you are eating the right meals for you. If you are starving within an hour or two, the previous meal was distinctly lacking. Keeping to these principles should enable you to experiment with the foods that keep you satisfied for longer.

2. Increase nutrient intake with juices and smoothies.

Base them on vegetables with small amounts of fruit. Smoothies can also include fats (coconut oil, avocado) and protein (nuts, seeds). For anyone looking to recover their health, these are a very beneficial way to boost nutrient intake and they are also efficient from a digestive viewpoint. This is even more so with a juice which enables you to absorb the vitamins straight away with minimal digestion. Frequency is an individual affair. For prevention you may be fairly inconsistent, but just know, when you do get around to making one, that it is very good for you! In recovery you may be more diligent, and some therapeutic diets include several juices each and every day.

3. Eliminate sugar and processed foods from your diet.

You can still have nice things, but just be discerning about quality. If sweet things are important to you, and you are not overweight, experiment with making your own cakes and biscuits out of high quality ingredients (pass on wheat flour and oils of questionable quality).

4. Include some raw foods with each meal.

Raw foods are packed with nutrients and contains live enzymes. Fine chopping makes raw food easier to digest. For instance, I might add some chopped raw broccoli to a Sunday roast, or serve bolognaise over a plate of raw courgette noodles (for which you will need a spiralizer – a fantastic gadget!) In Chinese Medicine raw foods have a cooling effect and help to clear heat and toxins. In contrast, cooked foods can be nourishing and warming, and so a balance is good.

5. Balance your plate

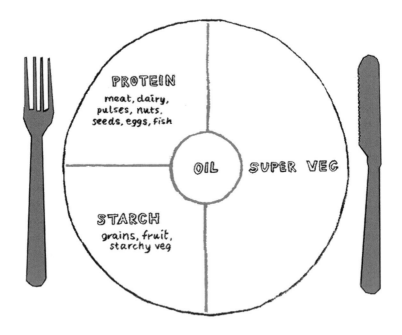

- Eat a rainbow diet – lots of colour comes from vegetables – all of which are teaming with nutrients to enhance how well your body functions

- Have protein with every meal

- Limit the starchy carbs – grains, root vegetables, and potato

- Include generous amounts of good fats, found in coconut oil, olive oil, nuts, seeds, avocado and coconut milk

6. Hydrate!

Drink lots of water and herbal or redbush teas. Green tea has anti-cancer properties[140] and 2-3 cups daily is recommended. Try different varieties, ginger green tea is one of my favourites. Go slow on caffeine, particularly if you are a slow metaboliser (it is very easy now to find this out from genetic testing – see Chapter Eight – or you might find that coffee makes your heart race, which would suggest you don't tolerate it well). Never use coffee to get you through the day, but if you are well balanced, then an occasional cup after a meal (preferably black) should not pose a problem. A cappuccino or latte counts as an occasional treat, and you can still do the 'meet for a coffee' thing, but maybe opt for a green or herbal tea instead.

The *Outsmart Cancer* Food Groups

Meat

Animal products are a complete and rich source of the dietary amino acids which are essential for repair and growth. They also provide B vitamins, particularly B12, which is often deficient in vegetarian diets, and the minerals iron and zinc. For many people, myself included, animal husbandry is a real issue, both from the point of view of animal welfare and also the resulting quality of the meat. If you can get it, meat from pasture fed animals is undoubtedly superior, particularly in respect of the fat content, which will be richer in the anti-inflammatory omega 3 than its intensively reared cousins, and also the beneficial fat called CLA (conjugated linoleic acid). Locally farmed or organic livestock are managed without the routine use of antibiotics or growth hormones, and have high standards of welfare, including access to the outdoors.[141] An animal spending a lifetime of grazing will be fitter and healthier, with undoubtedly lower stress hormones than one intensively reared. Hence, the meat quality and taste will be superior.

Dr Natasha Campbell-McBride is a Russian medical doctor who advocates a meat based diet for developmental and digestive issues. She advises that you should not only eat muscle meat, but also the organ meats that supply concentrated nutrients, including the valuable Co Enzyme Q10, which plays a role in cellular energy production. Organ meats have been enjoying a small revival, often referred to as 'nose to tail' dining. In years gone by, such culinary traditions would have been passed down through the generations, so that people had a taste for such foods and knew how to cook them. This is less true nowadays. Liver is a palatable food to begin your reintroduction to offal, and is often on the menu in good quality, family run Italian restaurants. Or it can be readily cooked at home, sautéed in butter with onions and mushrooms. Leftovers can be blended to make a well flavoured pate. In the UK, Waitrose sell organic chicken livers.

Of course locally sourced, high quality meat is more expensive, and for some people the budget can be an issue. There are ways around this. Some of the fattier cuts of meat, again from well farmed animals, make for lovely tasty stews and offer a less expensive option to the muscle meats. Offal is often a less expensive option too. Using smaller quantities alongside pulses and vegetables to add bulk can be a cost effective way of making family meals go further. It's not necessary to have meat every day and the budget can be balanced by offering a range of different protein foods within the diet.

From a health point of view, it is advisable to avoid processed meats like sausages and burgers, unless they come from a trusted source, such as a local farm shop or butcher, on the basis of the unknown levels of additives, preservatives and fillers that could be included. As Jamie Oliver showed us, there can be some quite unsavoury ingredients in a turkey twizzler!

Finally, bone broth is something to consider. If you are buying higher quality meat, then this is an excellent way to use all of the goodness, and to add taste to soups and stews. Bone broth is rich in minerals for bone and joint heath, such as magnesium and calcium, and in amino acids, such as glutamine, which benefits gut health too. It is very easy to make, especially if you use a slow cooker (see Chapter Six).

Fish

Fish and seafood are an easy to access and often fast to prepare meal choice. Think of prawns defrosted and added to a salad, a piece of wild salmon topped with pesto as a main course, or a grocery staple of tinned sardines or mackerel spread on wheat free toast or crackers.

Unless you live by the sea, fresh sources of local fish may be hard to come by and fish mongers are generally less prevalent than say, butchers. I tend to buy fish from the supermarket and generally look for those from sustainable sources. Wild salmon, if it's available, is a better choice than farmed varieties.

Fish, whether white or oily, is a light and digestible protein source. In addition, the oily fish such as salmon, trout, mackerel, sardines, herring and anchovies – have oil in their tissues as well as the liver, and their fillets can be up to 30% oil. The omega 3 content of fish oil is a powerful anti-inflammatory and therefore very health friendly. Omega 3 oils exert many anticancer actions that are crucial to preventing the onset and progression of cancer cells, including inhibiting cell proliferation, angiogenesis, metastasis and gene expression.[142] If you really don't like to eat fish, then you should consider taking fish oil supplements.

Smoked fish contains low levels of harmful polycyclic aromatic hydrocarbons (PAHs) as a residue from the smoking process, and this may pose an elevated cancer risk at high consumption rates over many years.[143] Personally, I do enjoy some smoked fish on occasion, but if you are in health recovery this is an avoidable toxin exposure that you could best do without.

Another consideration regarding fish consumption and health is the potential for heavy metal accumulation, including mercury.

Going up the food chain there can be a concentration of heavy metal pollutants in larger fish versus the smaller types that they feed on. This is why larger fish such as tuna and sword fish are best eaten in moderation, and a maximum intake of twice per month may be prudent.

Eggs & Dairy

Eggs are nature's ultimate fast food! They are a very high quality source of protein and relatively inexpensive – locally to us organic eggs are around 30p each. My favourite is to poach eggs in the steamer using egg pods that are widely available either in the supermarket or online. These are flexible silicon cooking cups, which can also be used for poaching in hot water (using the steamer is just a bit easier). Simply add a drop of oil and crack open the egg, and then place in the steamer until poached (around 5 to 10 minutes). Once cooked, use a knife to release the egg and then press it out onto either wheat-free toast or a salad.

Other ways to use eggs are in frittatas and a favourite in our house is to make it with sausage meat from the local farm shop. Scrambled eggs and omelettes are great for breakfasts and light meals, or you can make little egg muffins, which are popular with kids.

Used in baking, eggs also increase protein content and help to bind ingredients together. If you have an intolerance to eggs, then using ground flax seeds in baking is a good alternative.

I'm not as keen on fried eggs, as the higher cooking temperature is more likely to encourage oxidation of the cholesterol content. On that note, there is no evidence that eating eggs increases blood cholesterol levels, so don't let this be a reason to avoid them. Eggs also contain lecithin, which helps the digestion of fats and excretion of cholesterol. Lecithin is very brain friendly and helps to make the memory molecule, acetyl choline.

Earlier I discussed the pros and cons of dairy products (see Chapter Three). If you are in poor health, then avoiding dairy is a sensible option. There are now many types of non-dairy milk available. Good options are the various types of nut milk – almond and coconut for instance, or hemp. If you use soy, then always go for unsweetened organic. It is really easy to make your own nut milks and to do this all you need is a Nut Milk Bag from Amazon (see Resources). The benefit is that you just make the amount you need and it is free from stabilisers and additives.

There is a brand of coconut yoghurt available in health shops called Co-Yo. It's a little bit more expensive than regular yoghurt, but very nice. Even if you are avoiding milk, you may be ok with plain natural bio-yoghurt. Choose goat's or sheep's yoghurt if you prefer to avoid cow's products. Much of the lactose is converted by the beneficial bacteria, and Greek yoghurt is strained to remove the whey, which reduces lactose even more. This is why it is so creamy and yummy! Don't opt for low fat versions, as higher fat is not a problem in a healthy diet and is preferable to increasing sugars, often found in low fat varieties. Choosing a fruit flavour also increases the sugar content, so stick with plain and add your own fruit.

Generally, I find that goat's and sheep's cheese can be well tolerated by most people and this has the benefit of increasing the number of protein sources available, particularly if you really love cheese! As always though, we are looking for variety, so try to avoid over eating any one food group.

Although I've given cow's dairy the thumbs down, if you are lucky enough to obtain raw milk or cheese, then this can have positive health benefits. It is thought that the highly intensive management of cattle, and the processing of their milk, are responsible for its ill effects in many people. Raw milk is rich in natural enzymes (denatured by pasteurisation) which make it more easily digestible. It is also a source of the good bacteria which underpin good health. Because of potential health issues when milk is not pasteurised, raw milk production is tightly legislated and it is only available directly from the farm gate, or ordered online from registered suppliers (see Resources). The sale of raw milk is banned in Scotland.[144]

A further way to make milk more beneficial is to make kefir, a yoghurt-like drink made from adding milk to kefir grains (see Chapter Six). This is to reduce the lactose level and increases both probiotic and vitamin content, and is really easy to do at home.

Pulses

Pulses and beans are a valuable source of vegetarian protein, slow release carbohydrates and fibre. They are a good source of carotene (the precursor to vitamin A), vitamin E and the B vitamins, and the minerals potassium, calcium and magnesium.

Pulses add considerable convenience to a diet. They have a long shelf life and are a store cupboard staple; either in dried form, which requires some preparation, or from a tin or carton, where they are literally ready to eat. What could be easier than that? If you're not used to eating them then there may be a bit of a learning curve for trying out new dishes, so just don a positive attitude, reach for some recipes and give it a go.

As a form of protein, pulses are extremely economical and can help to balance the household budget, particularly when sourcing local farm raised meats and organic produce, which are relatively expensive. Whole meals can be replaced with vegetarian options several times a week, which increases variety too. Or pulses can be added to meat based dishes to add bulk and texture. For non-meat eaters, and particularly vegans, they are an essential form of protein, yet it is surprising how many vegetarians don't eat them regularly, preferring to bulk up on far less nutritious grains instead.

Some people may find that eating pulses and beans can make them a little windy, contribute to bloating or give digestive distress. This may indicate a need to improve digestion generally, such as by addressing stomach acid, digestive enzymes, or to improve the gut flora via probiotics (see Chapter Seven). Preparation can also help. Dry pulses usually need to be soaked prior to cooking (an exception to this is red lentils). Changing the soak water a couple of times can help to remove natural enzyme inhibitors and anti-nutrients like phytate.

A really terrific way to improve digestibility, nutrient availability and make them 'ready to eat' is to sprout beans and pulses. This is so easy to do, and bean sprouts are delicious. Just soak your chosen beans or seeds overnight, discard the soak water, rinse and drain. Repeat the rinsing process twice a day for 2-4 days until the sprouts are one to two inches long. Sprouting kits can be purchased on the internet, or made at home from a jam jar with a muslin lid. Once sprouted, keep them in an airtight pot in the fridge and add liberally to salads and cooked dishes.

Chick peas, mung beans and lentils are a good combination, and can be purchased as a dry sprouting mix or just use store bought already sprouted ones. Broccoli sprouts pack a powerful anticancer punch. A recent 12 week randomised control study in China found that detoxification was enhanced with a daily dose of a broccoli sprout derived beverage. The 291 study participants lived in an area characterized by exposure to substantial levels of airborne pollutants. The people eating the broccoli sprouts had significantly raised levels of pollutants in their urine compared to those without, meaning that the toxins were more efficiently excreted. In respect of airborne pollutants, which are associated with lung cancer and cardio-pulmonary disease, the authors conclude that broccoli sprouts utilised by people in high pollution areas "may provide a frugal means to attenuate their associated long-term health risks".[145]

Vegetables, Vegetables, Vegetables

Vegetables are arguably the most powerful weapon in your *Outsmart Cancer* arsenal. This is where a significant proportion of micronutrients – the vitamins, minerals and phytonutrients – come from. Vegetables add colour, variety and versatility to your meals. Chris Woollams of CancerActive has written a whole book about the rainbow diet and how it can help you beat cancer.[146] Government guidelines advise us to eat 5 portions of fruit and veg a day, which many experts find to be on the conservative side, and yet only 30% of the adult population in the UK achieve even this many.[147] So, for many people, there is significant room for improvement! Because veg is one of my main 'go to' foods, most days I can clock up 8 or 9 portions and that's without green juicing. This is easily done if you have 2 or 3 veg with each meal, including breakfast, and maybe as an odd snack too.

Of course, fresh juices are a fantastic way to massively increase your vegetable intake. By removing the fibre, the whole plant based goodness can easily be absorbed without requiring much effort at all from your digestive system and the nutrients can then flood into all the cells of your body. Smoothies and soups also make fast, satisfying and nutrient dense meals, which can pack several types of vegetable into one glass or bowl.

Non-starchy vegetables can be eaten freely and, in addition to being rich in micronutrients, contribute carbohydrate and a small amount of protein to your diet. These are predominantly 'above the ground' vegetables including green and salad varieties, and are listed in the shopping list table.

Starchy vegetables are often, but not exclusively, 'below the ground' vegetables, containing a higher carbohydrate content, which can rapidly increase blood glucose levels if eaten in quantity, therefore portion control is important. These vegetables include potato, sweet potato, butternut squash, carrots, parsnips, beetroot, peas and sweetcorn. Just have one selection of either starchy veg or grains (which are also starchy) and combine this with several non-starchy veg and protein per meal.

Whilst eating a wide array of vegetables is recommended, from an *Outsmart Cancer* perspective, ensure you include these within your diet:

- The cruciferous or brassica family, so named because their four petal arrangement resembles a cross. This includes cauliflower, cabbage, bok choi, Brussel sprouts, kale and collard greens. They contain a compound called glucosinolates that gives rise to compounds including indole-3-carbinole (I3C) and 3,3'-diindolylmethane (DIM), which support healthy oestrogen metabolism.[148]

- Mushrooms, particularly oriental varieties. In Chapter Two I considered the importance of mushrooms for immune health.

- The allium family – leeks, onions, garlic, chives and shallots. These are a source of sulphur molecules (along with eggs), which play an important role in detoxification. Onions and garlic are helpful for gut health.

- Tomatoes are an excellent source of lycopene, which is responsible for their red colour, and is more concentrated when cooked. It has been particularly studied in prostate cancer, where it is believed to exert an antioxidant effect.[149]

- Avocados are a real superfood, containing good fats and rich in nutrients including magnesium, potassium and B vitamins. They add a delectable creaminess to foods, particularly salads. You need not feel guilty eating avocados regularly, and they can even be added to smoothies to improve the texture.

Grains

Grains are cereal crops and include wheat, barley, rye, oats, rice and others. They are a dominant food group in the developed world today, and form the bulk of many food diaries that I see. I've already made a case for reducing or eliminating wheat in your diet (see Chapter Three) based on its poor nutrient content, high glycaemic index (it breaks down into glucose or sugar very quickly) and potentially allergenic profile. So that rules out regular bread for me; you may be able to get away with some, but don't let it dominate your meals.

Many people get on well with having some rye in their diet, either as rye bread or ryvita (but not coeliacs, as rye contains gluten). Because rye is quite dense, it doesn't tend to spike sugar levels quite as much as wheat. It can also be enjoyed as an open sandwich with vegetables and protein to make the overall meal more nutritious. Another option is sour dough bread, which is naturally fermented. This improves its digestibility.

Oats too are usually well tolerated, and can be eaten as granola or porridge. Oats can also be ground to make an oat flour for biscuits and pancakes.

If you are currently eating a lot of bread products, it may seem quite scary to think about giving them up. You just need to find another way to base your meals and use alternatives. With a little practice you'll discover a whole new world of eating.

Gluten free options may be a start, but also consider making a step change in reducing the amount of grains in your diet. So gluten free pasta with a meat and vegetable bolognaise may be a good choice, but a gluten free sandwich is still a sandwich. Could you swap it for a large salad or a bowl of soup? Alternatively make a wrap out of nori (seaweed), or even lettuce leaves – just pile in the filling and enjoy.

Nuts, seeds and oats can be ground into flour and used in baking - biscuits and cakes are not forbidden, but the ingredients should be healthy. Other alternative, non-gluten flours include gram flour (made from chickpeas), buckwheat, almond, coconut or quinoa. Rice and potato flours are also gluten free, but have a higher Glycaemic Load (GL).

I'm a big fan of the paleo diet, because it focuses on real food and cooking, and although going totally grain free can yield good results initially, on a prolonged basis it can also lead to becoming a little bit constipated. This is another reason you might prefer a mixed diet including both meat and pulses, but on the grains side I do think a small portion of rice on occasion can be helpful. Just settle for 3 or 4 tablespoons with protein and plenty of veg.

Back to the bolognaise sauce, a really great gadget is a spiralizer, which makes 'pasta' out of raw courgettes and other root vegetables. It's a fantastic invention and very popular with the children too. I once took one into a primary school for a demonstration of child friendly foods and the teachers were amazed that even some of their renowned fussy eaters really enjoyed courgette noodles! Another alternative for you is kelp noodles, online or from a health shop, which are made from sea weed.

Are you familiar with quinoa? This is technically a seed, not a grain, but is used like cous cous (which is wheat based). Quinoa takes around 15 minutes to cook, but can also be purchased pre-cooked in packets (Merchant Gourmet, usually located in the pulses section). It really picks up flavours well, and can make a stand alone vegetarian meal, with added pulses and vegetables.

Fruit

As part of a cancer protection diet, fruit is really nutritious, providing heaps of vitamins and fibre. It is also convenient and portable, and makes for a handy snack or desert after a meal. Personally I like to add some fruit to salads to give them a million dollar taste. Some of my favourites are prawn & mango, chicken & papaya or some plain chopped apple with red cabbage. I've even added some fresh, chopped pineapple to a cooked breakfast of bacon and eggs at a networking meeting, which drew a few inquisitive glances!

Some people have heard about food combining, which suggests that fruit shouldn't be eaten with any other food. Try for yourself, but my clients regularly mix fruit with or after meals and don't have any problems. Maybe if people are eating lots of grains and pasta (which I don't advocate) then food combining may be a bigger issue, as these foods tend to be stodgier. There is an advantage in eating fruit alongside meals containing fat and protein which digest more slowly and thus temper the release of sugar from the fruit.

Because fruit is quite high in fructose, a natural sugar, it is sensible to limit portions and two to three pieces a day is optimal. When using a larger piece of fruit, say a mango, simply cut off a chunk and return the remainder to the fridge in an airtight container for another day. It keeps quite well and then there's not the pressure to eat the whole thing in one sitting. Lower sugar options are berries of any type – blueberry, strawberry, blackberry, raspberry - and cherries. Some fruits are quite high in sugar and it is best to avoid eating them on their own, unless you are doing a lot of physical activity. These include bananas, grapes and dried fruit like sultanas. They can however be used in small quantities in baking or smoothies where they can add a natural sweetness, and the accompanying fat and protein slows down their glycaemic impact.

Nuts and Seeds

Unless you have allergies, nuts and seeds are a terrific source of good fats, protein and nutrients such as calcium, magnesium and vitamin E.

With the exception of chestnuts, nuts are high in fat, moderate in protein and low in carbs which is an excellent profile for our purposes. Almonds and cashews contain slightly higher protein, whilst coconut, brazil nuts and macadamias have a higher fat content:

Per 100g dry weight	Protein	Fat	Carbs
Almond	22	58	7
Brazil	14	70	3

Cashew	21	52	6
Chestnut	4	6	76
Coconut	6	71	7
Hazelnut	15	66	6
Macadamia	8	76	4
Pine nut	14	70	4
Walnut	15	70	3

Source: The Composition of Foods (1993)

The fats in most nuts and seeds are predominantly omega 6 polyunsaturated and monounsaturated fat. However, flax and chia seeds deserve special mention, along with walnuts, as they are rich sources of the anti-inflammatory omega 3 oils.

Seeds are, on average, higher in protein, lower in fat and higher in carbohydrate than nuts. They are an excellent source of minerals and contain high levels of potassium, calcium, magnesium, iron and zinc. The mineral composition of wholemeal wheat flour is shown for comparison:

Mg per 100g dry weight	**Potassium**	**Calcium**	**Magnesium**	**Iron**	**Zinc**
Pumpkin	880	46	584	16	8
Sesame	597	702	388	11	6
Sunflower	743	115	408	7	5
Flax	831	236	431	5	4
Wholemeal wheat flour	395	44	140	4	3

Source: The composition of food. FSA. (3rd edition)

Now you can see why seeds are considered to be superfoods!

Using nut and seed flours is a really nutritious way to transition into healthier eating. I have already mentioned UGG foods – who offer paleo style bread and cake mixes - no grains, no dairy, no added sugar (see Resources). You can buy the packet mixes online and quickly knock up a feast just by adding eggs and oil. UGG use chia seed and almond flour, which give a beautifully dense texture and are filling too.

You can also make your own bread, cakes and crackers from nuts, seeds and oat flour. The flax seed focaccia is a firm favourite and very good for soluble fibre. Not to be missed is my chocolate brownie recipe – decadent, delicious and good for you too (see Chapter Five)!

Because of the high polyunsaturated fat content of nuts and seeds, they easily become rancid. If you have the fridge space, consider storing them in glass jars in the refrigerator to prolong their freshness. This is especially important if you buy ground flax seeds.

And finally, if you have digestive issues or eat a lot of nuts and seeds, you may benefit from soaking them for a few hours or overnight. This helps to reduce the naturally occurring phytic acid content which can inhibit mineral absorption, and it also neutralises enzyme inhibitors. Either drain and rinse them ready for use, or dry them for storage in a dehydrator (see Resources), cool oven or by leaving them for a period in a warm airing cupboard.

Oils

For cooking, use saturated fats, such as coconut oil, butter or solid forms including duck or goose fat, as these are stable at high temperatures. Olive oil, which is a monounsaturated oil can also be heated gently or used cold in salads. Purchase olive oil in dark coloured glass bottles to protect it against oxidation.

Specialist, nut and seed oils such as cold pressed walnut, sesame and avocado oils are also good to use in salads, but don't heat them, as they are prone to oxidation. Personally, I wouldn't use any of the more commercial sunflower or corn oils. In addition to being unstable at temperature, their extraction processes often include heat and chemicals.

As previously discussed, as a spread, choose butter, not margarine. If you are lactose intolerant, then ghee, which can be purchased in jars or made at home, may be a better choice. To make ghee, heat a pack of butter in a saucepan and once melted pass it through a muslin to remove the milk solids and protein. The resulting clear liquid quickly solidifies and can be refrigerated.

Flax seed oil, which is a rich source of omega 3, has been shown to have anti-carcinogenic properties, particularly with hormonally based tumours. In animal studies, flax oil was found to enhance the tumour reducing effects of Trastuzumab (Herceptin).[150] A further study using mice with ER positive breast tumours recorded a reduction in tumour size (-33%), cell proliferation (-38%) and an increase in apoptosis (+10%).[151]

Dr Johanna Budwig, a German biochemist and expert on fatty acids, developed the Budwig protocol in 1952 as an anti-cancer therapy. She advocated that healthy people should take 1 tbsp of flax oil daily, and in sickness this should increase to 6-8 tbsp. The oil should be combined thoroughly into either quark, cottage cheese or plain natural yoghurt and left to stand for 10 minutes to allow the fatty acids to interact with the protein. As flax oil is very unstable, it should at least be refrigerated after opening and, if possible, kept in the deep freeze. It has a low melting point and will melt at room temperature within minutes.

Herbs and Spices

Herbs and spices add colour and taste to meals, but did you know that some can also have healing properties?

The most well known in the cancer field is turmeric, the bright yellow spice most often used in South Asian and Middle Eastern cuisine. The active ingredient within turmeric is curcumin, and this has powerful antioxidant and anti-inflammatory properties. It is one of the ten supplements discussed in a review by the Society of Integrative Oncology,[152] who quote:

"Curcumin has been shown to prevent a large number of cancers in animal studies. Laboratory data indicate that curcumin can inhibit tumour initiation, promotion, invasion, angiogenesis, and metastasis."

Turmeric, or curcumin, can be taken as a supplement of course. But it can also be useful in cooking, imparting a gentle golden colour, and is frequently used alongside other spices to create a curry flavour.

Cinnamon is a warming spice, which is also high in antioxidants and has a history of use in helping to improve blood sugar regulation and insulin sensitivity, which in turn may be beneficial for reducing cancer risk.

Generally feel that you can use herbs and spices liberally in the kitchen. If you are able to grow some of your own herbs you'll have a ready supply and the freshness of picking when you need it.

Sweeteners

As cancer cells are sugar hungry, you will obviously want to limit your sugar intake. This could also protect you from other chronic health conditions like heart disease and dementia, as the inflammation arising from high blood sugar levels is a factor in many modern chronic diseases.

However, to make cakes and desserts, you will need to add some sweetness to your baking. Consider using fruit such as mashed banana, apples and even carrots. Dried fruit too can be useful in small amounts.

There are a number of sweeteners on the market. Xylitol or stevia are recommended.

Xylitol is a sugar alcohol which occurs naturally in fruits and vegetables; industrially it is extracted from birch trees. It imparts a sweetness without affecting blood sugar levels, is without a bitter aftertaste and has an excellent safety profile. One study over two years showed no ill effects. The only potential downside is that over consumption could lead to diarrhoea. Please note though that xylitol is toxic to dogs, so keep baking well away from any pets.

Stevia is another natural sweetener that has gained in popularity. Some people find it has a bitter after taste.

I encourage you not to use artificial sweeteners. Aspartame is potentially associated with many side effects, including headaches, heart palpitations and joint pain. One study comparing participants on a high vs low aspartame diet of 8 days duration noted more irritable mood and depression associated with aspartame consumption.[153]

In the past, agave nectar or syrup was promoted as healthy due to its low GI. However more recently there has been concern that it contains high levels of fructose, which is potentially associated with non-alcoholic fatty liver disease.

If you are in good health, then you may prefer to use small amounts of natural sweetness, such as local raw honey (which has many other health benefits including healing and antibacterial properties), maple syrup or blackstrap molasses. However, these do contain both sucrose and fructose and will elevate blood sugar levels, so use sparingly.

The *Outsmart Cancer* Shopping List

Use this guide to plan your new eating regime. You can print the shopping list online at www.OutsmartCancer.co.uk, where you will find different versions for vegetarian and paleo diets.

PROTEIN – animal based Organic or farm raised where possible	Poultry - chicken, turkey etc. Meat – Venison, Lamb, beef, pork etc. Organ meats such as liver are beneficial. No processed meats Eggs No Cow's dairy. Occasional goat's or sheep's cheese, depending on your individuality
PROTEIN – seafood	Fish – Salmon, mackerel, trout, cod, seabass, tuna, plaice etc. Other – prawns, scallops, etc.
PROTEIN – vegetarian (Pulses only if you have good digestion)	Lentils - puy, beluga, red, green Beans - red kidney, cannellini, butter bean, chick peas, etc. Peas – yellow split Tofu, soy, oyster & shitake mushrooms
SUPER VEG Eat generously	Artichoke, Asparagus, Aubergine, Avocado, Bean sprouts, Broccoli, Brussels Sprouts, Cabbage, Cauliflower, Celeriac, Celery, Courgettes, Cucumbers, Fennel, Garlic, Green beans, Kale, Kohlrabi, Lettuce, Leeks, Mooli, Mushrooms,

	Olives, Onions, Peppers, Pumpkin, Rocket, Salad greens, Spinach, Sprouts, String Beans, Tomatoes, Watercress
STARCH With every meal but limit portion	Veg (max 100g) - carrots, parsnip, sweet potato, beetroot, butternut squash, peas, sweetcorn Quinoa, Oats, Brown rice, Millet, Buckwheat, Potato, No wheat
FRUIT 2-3 pieces daily	Apples, Apricots, Blackberries, Blueberries, Cherries, Grapefruit, Kiwi Fruit, Lemons, Limes, Mango, Melon, Oranges, Papaya, Peaches, Plums, Pomegranate, Nectarine, Raspberries, Strawberries etc. No bananas, grapes or dried fruit, unless used in baking or smoothies
OILS	For cooking – only Butter, Coconut Oil or Olive Oil. Other cold pressed oils can be used cold (eg: Flax, Walnut, Sesame) Nuts: Almonds, Brazil, Cashew, Coconut, Walnut etc. Can be used to make milk and nut butters Seeds: Chia, Hemp, Flax, Pumpkin, Sesame, Sunflower

Additional Items

FLOUR	Corn flour (in small amounts eg: to thicken gravy). Nut flours: almond, and coconut, flax seeds, quinoa flour, buckwheat flour
VINEGAR	Apple cider (preferred), balsamic, wine vinegar
FLAVOURINGS	Bouillon powder (I use Marigold) Sea salt Tamari (wheat free soy sauce) Mustard – all types Tahini – ground sesame paste Pesto Curry paste
BAKING	Good quality vanilla extract 70% dark chocolate
HERBS (fresh or dried)	Herbes de Provence, oregano, chilli, rosemary, mint, coriander, parsley etc.
SPICES	Cinnamon, cumin, curry powder, coriander, turmeric, paprika, nutmeg, 5 spice, jerk

Summary

The *Outsmart Cancer* eating plan is a change to your lifestyle, where real unprocessed natural foods take centre stage. You need not go hungry, as portions can be plentiful.

1. Try to balance each meal with protein, lots of veg, fruit, oil or fat and starch. Limit starchy carbohydrate intake and keep sugar intake to an absolute minimum.

2. You can have occasional treats, particularly if you are in good health, but try to be discerning about quality. Making your own can be very satisfying.

3. Spend some time transitioning to your healthier regime, and know that this will soon become a new habit, which with a little planning, will be quick and easy to follow.

Above all, enjoy your food! Next we'll look at recipes to give you a head start.

Chapter Five:
Food, Glorious Food!

Now that I have established why nutrition is so important for health, and broadly what to eat, it is time to embark on recipes to entice you into your new regime.

In a way, recipes are usually never in short supply, as most of us tend to have several cookbooks on our shelves. TV cooking shows, and recipes in magazines and on the internet abound. The challenge lies in translating new ideas off the page or screen and into your kitchen.

So this chapter aims to give you a head start. I encourage you to read through and if something takes your fancy, commit to adding the ingredients to your next shopping list.

Also keep an eye out for new recipes via the website www.OutsmartCancer.co.uk, and consider following us on Facebook.

Here you will find several recipes for each major eating segment – breakfast, light meals, sides, main meals, bread & crackers, sweet treats and drinks, smoothies & juices.

Breakfast

Broccoli Guacamole with Poached Egg & Sundried Tomatoes - Serves 2

Bright & colourful, this is a powerful way to pack in a couple of vegetable portions at the start of your day. German rye bread can be purchased from either a supermarket or a local baker; and the recipe for flax bread (which is gluten free) follows.

Ingredients

2 eggs
4 broccoli florets, cooked
1 avocado
2 tbsp soft goat's cheese, or olive oil if you are dairy free
4 sundried tomatoes
Flax or rye bread
S&P

Method

1. Poach the eggs. I use an electric steamer – adding the eggs to a silicon poach pod and steaming for 8-10 minutes.

2. Add the broccoli, avocado and goat's cheese or oil to a small blender and whizz until smooth. Check the consistency and add a dash of hot water if required. Give a final whizz.

3. Spread the guacamole over a slice of flax or rye bread and top with the sundried tomatoes.

4. Loosen the egg in the pod by running a knife around the outside. Cut a criss cross pattern and pop out over the tomatoes.

Chocolate Chia Porridge - Serves 1

A variation on traditional porridge using the superfood, chia seeds. Like flax, chia seeds are mucilagenic and readily absorb water which can be very helpful for keeping you regular. This recipe has a touch of luxury with the sweetness of apple and a creamy chocolatey flavour.

Ingredients

20g chia seeds
Handful of almonds – soaked in water for 4 – 8 hours or overnight
1 cup warm water
1 apple (cored and chopped – leave skin on)
1 tsp raw cacao (or organic cocoa powder
Pinch of cinnamon & a tsp of flaked coconut (optional)

Method

1. Steam the apple for 5 minutes.

2. Drain and rinse the almonds. Blend almonds, apple, cacao and water. Add more water if required to achieve a thick but runny consistency.

3. Pour over the chia seeds, stir well and leave for anywhere between 15 minutes and overnight.

4. Sprinkle with cinnamon and top with coconut flakes to serve.

Breakfast Pancakes - Serves 4

A nourishing way to start to the day. These pancakes are fairly time consuming to make, so are best tackled when you have more time such as over the weekend. The mixture keeps in the fridge for up to 3 days.

When adding the mixture, add enough to generously cover the bottom of the pan. If you find that the pancakes break, then make them slightly thicker and leave to cook for slightly longer, so that they are a toasted brown colour.

Ingredients

75g ground almonds
50g oats, ground to a flour-like consistency
2 eggs
300ml nut milk (eg: almond, coconut)
Glug of olive oil plus oil for frying (coconut is best)
S&P

Method

1. Add the ground almonds, oats, eggs, milk, salt and oil to a blender and blitz.

2. Heat the coconut oil in a small frying pan and add half a ladle full of mixture. Heat through until the mixture sets and then flip over to cook the other side.

3. Stack the pancakes as you make them. Serve with plain goat's yoghurt and fresh fruit.

Mel's Almond Granola - Serves 10

I was introduced to this delicious home-made granola when staying with Melanie Gamble, from the charity Together Against Cancer. This makes about 10 generous portions. Although it does contain maple syrup as a natural sweetener, this works out at less than a teaspoon per portion. The high protein and fat content slows down the release of sugar, and so this is a breakfast that should keep you fuller for longer.

Ingredients

2.5 cups oats
1 cup shredded coconut
1 cup whole almonds
45ml or 3 tbsp maple syrup
¼ cup almond butter
Generous ¼ cup coconut oil

Method

1. Preheat oven to 190°C.

2. In a small pan, melt the coconut oil, maple syrup and almond butter.

3. Stir in the dry ingredients and mix well. Turn out onto a shallow baking tray and bake for 20 – 30 minutes or until crispy.

4. Once cooled, store in an airtight container.

Light Meals

Red Lentil Soup – Serves 2

This warming soup is a terrific standby as it uses predominantly store cupboard ingredients. Add a generous grind of black pepper, which helps to increase the absorption of curcumin, the active ingredient in turmeric.

Ingredients

170g red lentils
450ml cold water
2 tsp bouillon
1 carrot, scrubbed and chopped
1 onion, peeled and sliced
2 cloves of garlic, minced
1/2 inch of ginger, finely chopped
1 tsp turmeric
1 tsp mild curry powder
1 tbsp Coconut oil
400ml hot water or stock
S&P

Method

1. Rinse the lentils and place them in a saucepan with the bouillon and water. Bring to the boil, cover and simmer gently for 20 mins.

2. Sauté the vegetables, garlic and spices in coconut oil until they are soft.

3. Mix the vegetables into the lentils and place in a high speeder blender with the hot water or stock – blend until creamy. Adjust to the desired consistency by adding water, check the seasoning and serve.

Cashew and Spinach Soup – Serves 2

This soup is always a real hit in workshops, and is especially fast to make.

To roast the butternut squash, score the skin and bake it whole for around 40 minutes in a hot oven (200 degrees). Cool and refrigerate until it is ready to use. Roasted squash makes an excellent base to soups and can be added to casseroles. Simply slice as required, and discard the seeds and skin.

Ingredients

1 tbsp coconut oil (optional)
1 large onion, roughly chopped
2 cloves garlic, chopped
60g cashew nuts
2 tsp bouillon
150g roasted butternut squash
2 tbsp of thick coconut milk (from a tin)
500ml hot water
2 large handfuls of spinach
S&P

Method

1. Steam or sauté the onions and garlic in coconut oil until soft.

2. Add the cashews and bouillon to a blender, blitz into a powder.

3. Add the onions, garlic, butternut squash, coconut cream and hot water to the blender. Whizz until smooth.

4. Add the spinach, then blend once again until smooth. Serve in a large mug or soup bowl.

Mediterranean Vegetable Frittata – Serves 4 to 6

This is a very flexible dish where you can simply add any vegetables that you like. A shortcut would be to reuse some left over roasted vegetables, then simply add the beaten eggs, season and bake.

The recipe also lends itself to mini Mediterranean muffins – here you can use a muffin tray and divide the mixture between individual muffin cases. In this case check them after 20 minutes as they cook more quickly.

Ingredients

1 red pepper, sliced into long strips
1 red onion, chopped
1 courgette, sliced
200g button mushrooms, sliced
2 cloves of garlic, crushed
1 tbsp. coconut oil
1 large sweet potato, peeled, cubed and steamed until soft
8 eggs
S&P

Method

1. Preheat the oven to 200°C.

2. Saute the vegetables in the coconut oil until softened. Place them in a shallow casserole dish.

3. Beat the eggs, season to taste and pour over the vegetables.

4. Bake for 30 minutes and serve with a mixed salad and / or sauerkraut (see Chapter Six).

Jerk Chicken Salad - Serves 4

The combination of warm chicken with the crunchiness of salad vegetables and the sweetness of pineapple is an interesting combination. This is a substantial dish which is elegant enough to serve visitors for lunch, and convenient enough to be a family staple too.

Ingredients

1 tbsp olive oil
1 tbsp jerk seasoning
450g skinless chicken thighs, cut into strips
1 large romaine lettuce
½ medium pineapple, diced
1 red pepper thinly sliced
3 inch cucumber, diced
1 can red kidney beans
1 lime
100ml plain goats or soy yoghurt
2 tsp honey, or 1 tsp xylitol

Method

1. Preheat the oven to 200°C.

2. In a bowl, mix the jerk seasoning and olive oil. Add the chicken and mix well to coat the chicken.

3. Bake the chicken for 30 minutes, or until cooked.

4. Wash and shred the lettuce, use it to line a salad bowl.

5. Mix the pineapple, red pepper and cucumber through the lettuce. Add the kidney beans and mix well.

6. To make the dressing, zest the lime and add 1 tsp to the yoghurt along with the juice of half the fruit. Mix well and stir in honey to taste.

7. Add the hot chicken to the salad, top with dressing and mix well.

Sides

Courgette Coleslaw - Serves 4

Coleslaw is a great addition to a meal, and is very easy to make at home. You can vary the ingredients depending on the vegetables that you have available. This recipe works just as well with sweet potato or butternut squash to replace the carrot, or cabbage instead of courgette. A mandolin with a julienne blade is a useful investment to make coleslaw, or you could grate or finely chop the vegetables by hand or with a food processor instead.

Ingredients

1 large carrot
1 large courgette
1 red onion
1 tbsp pine nuts (optional)
1 tbsp mayonnaise or olive oil
2-3 tbsp plain goats or soy yoghurt
Fresh parsley to garnish (optional)

Method

1. Using the mandolin, julienne the courgette and carrot into matchsticks. Then finely chop the onion. Place the vegetables in a bowl.

2. Add the pine nuts if you are using them.

3. Add the mayonnaise or oil and yoghurt to the bowl, then season. Mix well to combine all of the ingredients. Sprinkle with chopped parsley and serve.

Cauliflower Rice - Serves 3 to 4

Cauliflower is the new star of the low carb world. Here it is made into a rice alternative, which can also be served raw. In this recipe, though, it is gently tossed in coconut oil. Another great advantage is that it is really, really superfast.

Ingredients

1 head of cauliflower
1-2 tbsp coconut oil

Method

1. Wash and dry the cauliflower, and cut into florets.

2. Place in small batches into a food processor and whizz for just a few seconds until you have achieved a 'rice' like consistency.

3. Gently melt the coconut oil in a frying pan. Toss the cauliflower in the oil until just warmed through, then serve.

Sweet Potato Chips - Serves 4

Sweet potato has a lower glycaemic index than regular potato, and adds a significant dose of vitamin A or beta-carotene. These are a much healthier alternative than regular oven chips!

Ingredients

3 large or 4 regular sized sweet potatoes, peeled
2 tbsp coconut oil
S&P

Method

1. Preheat the oven to 200 degrees.

2. Place the coconut oil in a baking tray and pop in the oven to melt whilst you prepare the potato.

3. Cut the sweet potato into chunky chips.

4. Using an oven glove, carefully remove the baking tray and toss the sweet potato in the warm oil. Season generously.

5. Bake for 30- 40 minutes or until soft on the inside and lightly crispy on the outside, and then serve.

Mashed Celeriac - Serves 4

Another low carb wonder, the humble celeriac is a delicious vegetable. This gives all of the comfort of mash, but again has a much lower glycaemic index.

Ingredients

One celeriac, peeled and roughly chopped
A generous knob of butte
1 tsp wholegrain mustard, or more to taste
S&P

Method

1. Either steam or gently simmer the celeriac in hot water until soft. Drain.

2. Add the butter and mustard.

3. Either mash by hand or use a food processor to blend the celeriac to a creamy consistency. Season to taste and serve.

Mains

Satay Noodles - Serves 2

This is a wonderfully nutritious, wheat free option to regular noodles. I first made it when working with a young University student with Ulcerative Colitis. This gave her a delicious alternative to the regular student fayre of lots of pasta, and at the same time enabled her to be a trend setter too.

Ingredients

1 large courgette
1 sliced yellow pepper
100g mange tout, steamed
100g of mixed bean sprouts (eg: aduki, lentil, chick pea, mung)
1 tbsp sesame seeds
2 tbsp tamari
120g almond butter
2 tbsp melted coconut oil
Squeeze of lemon
Pinch of chilli flakes

Method

1. Spiralize the courgette to make noodles (or use a julienne knife or mandolin) - see Chapter Six.

2. Place the courgette noodles, pepper, mange tout, bean sprouts and sesame seeds in a bowl. Mix well.

3. In a small pan, melt the coconut oil and add the almond butter, tamari, lemon juice and chilli flakes. Stir well to mix them into a smooth dressing and pour over the vegetables.

4. Mix well and serve.

Pesto Baked Salmon with Celeriac Mash - Serves 4

Oily fish contributes protein and the essential omega 3, which is anti-inflammatory and vital for brain health. The recipe here assumes you will make your own pesto, but if this is a push simply use a jar of ready-made pesto.

Ingredients

4 salmon fillets
50g pine nuts
Large bunch of basil
50 g grated parmesan
1 clove of garlic
150ml olive oil
8 cherry tomatoes
4 portions of celeriac mash (see previous)

Method

1. Preheat the oven to 190°C.

2. Lightly toast the pine nuts in a frying pan until slightly coloured (optional)

3. Blend the pine nuts, basil, garlic and parmesan by pulsing in a food processor. Gradually add the olive oil and continue to blend until smooth.

4. Place the salmon fillets on a baking tray and generously top with the pesto. Add the cherry tomatoes to the tray.

5. Bake for 20 minutes and serve with celeriac mash and green vegetables.

6. Return any leftover pesto to a glass jar and refrigerate for up to 2 weeks.

Chicken & Mango curry with Cauliflower 'Rice' - Serves 4

A creamy chicken curry with a subtle fruit flavour. Although the coriander isn't essential, it does finish the dish off nicely, and adds another boost of nutrients including vitamin A, vitamin C and potassium.

Ingredients

2 tbsp olive oil
500g chicken off the bone and cubed, thigh has the better flavour
1 large onion, peeled and sliced
2 cloves garlic, peeled and minced
1 inch ginger, peeled and minced
1 tsp medium curry powder
1 tsp turmeric
Half a tin of tomatoes
1 red pepper, diced
1 tsp bouillon powder
Dash of water as required
1 tin coconut milk
½ medium mango, diced
2 tbsp chopped coriander
4 portions of cauliflower rice (see previous)

Method

1. Saute the chicken in oil until it is lightly browned, then remove it to a plate.

2. Add the onions, garlic, ginger and spices to the pan with a little oil and saute with the spices.

3. Add the tomatoes and red pepper, with bouillon. Return the chicken to the pan.

4. Stir in the coconut milk. Lightly simmer for 20-30 minutes until cooked through. Add water as required.

5. Stir through the mango and top with coriander.

6. Serve with cauliflower rice and a green salad.

Vegetarian option – replace the chicken with chick peas or other pulses.

Bread & Crackers

Flax Seed Focaccia - Serves 6 to 8

This has the consistency of a cross between a bread and a savoury cake, and is my preferred non-gluten option. The flax seeds add fibre, protein and omega 3 plus a wealth of minerals.

Ingredients
240ml flax seed (also called linseed)
100ml oats or almond flour
2 tsp baking powder
½ tsp salt
3 eggs
85ml water
50ml olive oil
Tbsp pumpkin seeds

Method
1. Preheat the oven to 190°C.

2. Grind the flax and oats (or almond flour) in a high speed blender or coffee grinder to achieve the consistency of flour.

3. Add the baking powder and salt, then whizz briefly to blend.

4. Place the dry ingredients in a mixing bowl (you can, if you wish, store the mix at this point).

5. Add the eggs, oil and water to the dry ingredients and mix well.

6. Spread onto an oiled baking tray to a size of 9" x 8" (the size of a Pampered Chef small bar pan).

7. Sprinkle with pumpkin seeds and bake for 20 minutes.

8. Serve as a gluten free bread alternative.

Gram Flour Wraps - Serves 4

These little wraps are perfect for making fast lunches or a snack. Gram flour is made from chick peas and the resulting wraps are high in protein, nutritious and naturally gluten free.

Ingredients

200g gram flour
500ml water
¼ tsp turmeric
¼ tsp cayenne pepper
¼ tsp salt
Generous sprinkling of ground pepper

Method

1. Combine the dry ingredients in a bowl.

2. Add half the water and mix well with a whisk. Then add the rest of the water and continue to mix until it forms a smooth batter.

3. Set aside the batter for about 20 minutes. To make the wraps, use a small frying pan or crepe pan. Start by heating a ¼ tsp of coconut oil in the pan. Repeat this for each wrap.

4. Use a ladle to add the batter to the pan, aiming for a thin coating and gently shake to spread it evenly around.

5. Once the batter has started to dry on the top and the edges start to lift slightly, flip the wrap and cook for about 40 seconds.

6. Stack the wraps and store them in the refrigerator or use immediately.

7. To serve, top with a filling and roll into a sausage shape. Use whichever fillings take your fancy. For example – spread hummus with grated carrot, a sprinkling of sesame seeds and a squeeze of lemon juice.

Flax Seed Crackers

If you sometimes crave the comfort of carbiness, these are a delicious low carb and wheat free alternative to regular crackers. They are full of protein, fibre and minerals, and are ideal with dips and spreads.

Ingredients

1 cup flax seeds
1 cup sunflower seeds
1 tbsp sesame
½ red pepper
2 sun dried tomato
120ml water
½ tsp salt
1 egg

Method

1. Pre heat the oven to 150 degrees

2. Place the flax and sunflower seeds in a blender, and blitz into a flour like consistency.

3. Pour the 'flour' into a mixing bowl. Add the sesame seeds.

4. Place the red pepper, tomatoes, water and salt n the blender. Blitz briefly until the vegetables are finely chopped. Pour into the mixing bowl.

5. Add the egg, and mix well until the mixture forms a dough.

6. Split the dough into two, and spread thinly on two lightly oiled baking trays. I use Pampered Chef stoneware.

7. Using a knife, run lines down and across the flattened dough to make cracker shapes.

8. Bake for 35 minutes and then leave to cool in the oven. Once cooled keep in an airtight container in the fridge.

Sweet Treats

Chocolate Brownies - Serves 16

This delicious recipe is easy to make, gluten free and packed with protein from ground almonds, walnuts and eggs. And because it is so satisfying, you'll be less likely to over indulge too. A little bit of what you fancy can indeed do you good!

Ingredients

150g coconut oil or butter
90g honey
125g 70% chocolate
2 ripe bananas
2 tsp vanilla extract
4 eggs
2 tsp baking powder
30g cocoa powder
150g ground almonds
200g walnuts, chopped

Method

1. Pre heat the oven to 180°C.

2. Cream the oil or butter and sugar using a wooden spoon or mixer.

3. Melt the chocolate in a bowl over hot water or in a steamer.

4. Mash the bananas with the vanilla extract.

5. Beat the eggs in a bowl.

6. Mix the dry ingredients in a large bowl - almonds, baking powder, cocoa and walnuts.

7. Add the wet ingredients to the dry, stir to combine well. Pour into the lined cake tin and bake for 20- 25 minutes.

Baked Peaches & Coconut Cream - Serves 4

The chopped nuts give a crunchiness which contrasts well with the softness of the baked fruit. Coconut cream gives this desert a decadent finish.

Ingredients

4 peaches, halved and pitted
50g butter
30g coconut sugar or xylitol
100g chopped mixed nuts
1 tin of Coconut milk
1 tsp honey (optional)

Method

1. Melt the butter in a pan, stir in the coconut sugar or xylitol and then mix in the nuts.

2. Spoon the nut mixture into the peach halves. Place them in an ovenproof dish, cut surface uppermost.

3. Bake at 190°C for 15 minutes.

4. To make the coconut cream: refrigerate a tin of coconut cream for 24 hours.

5. Usually the tin of coconut milk separates. Place the thick coconut cream and light coconut water into a blender, add the honey (if using) and whip until light and creamy. Serve with the baked peaches.

Healthy Truffles - Serves 12

Good enough to treat! These truffles are packed full of nutrients and taste delicious too.

Ingredients

160g mixed seeds (flax, sunflower, pumpkin, sesame)
1 tbsp coconut oil
120g dried fruit (prunes and apricots or dates)
Cocoa powder or desiccated coconut (unsweetened)

Method

1. Grind the seeds to a powder, then transfer them to a mixing bowl.

2. Melt the coconut oil in a bain marie (or use a glass bowl in an electric steamer).

3. Add the oil and dried fruit to a blender. Blitz to a paste and then scrape the paste into a bowl.

4. Stir into the ground seeds; mix well.

5. Scoop into teaspoon sized balls, roll in cocoa powder or coconut and place in petit four cases.

6. Chill for a couple of hours and serve after a meal or as a snack.

Drinks

Strawberry Smoothie - Serves 1

Lecithin is derived from soy, and is a rich source of choline and phospholipids which are essential for brain health. It is available in health food shops, and gives an additional creaminess to this smoothie. Just a small amount of banana improves the consistency and adds a natural sweetness. Simply peel and freeze the remaining half for another day.

Ingredients

50g or a small handful of almonds, soaked overnight & drained
½ banana
Handful of strawberries
1 tsp lecithin (optional)

Method

1. Make a nut milk by rinsing the soaked almonds and placing them in a blender with 200ml fresh water. Blitz and then use a nut milk bag to separate the sediment (this can be used in baking and can be frozen until ready to use).

2. Return the nut milk to the blender with banana, fruit and lecithin (if using).

3. Blitz again until smooth and serve over ice.

Lemon & Gingerade - Serves 2

For the times when you are looking for a perkier drink than plain water, here is a recipe to add a healthy sparkle.

Ingredients

Juice of 1 lemon
1 inch of ginger (peeled & grated)
440ml coconut water
500ml fizzy water
Ice cubes
Fruit to garnish

Method

1. Add the lemon juice, ginger and coconut water to a jug.

2. Stir in the coconut water.

3. Top up with fizzy water, adding ice as required.

4. Decorate with slices of lemon, cucumber and /or strawberries.

Superpower Green Juice - Serves 2

Juices can be any combination of vegetables, with a small amount of fruit to add some sweetness. They are a concentrated source of nutrients which easily pass through your digestive system and into your cells.

Ingredients

1 green apple
½ cucumber
2 celery sticks
2 handfuls spinach
½ lemon

Method

1. Scrub the apple and salad vegetables well, and rinse the spinach.

2. Pass through a juicer, alternating hard items like apple with a few of the spinach leaves.

3. Add ice to serve (optional).

Red Beauty - Serves 2

Beetroot has an earthy taste and supports liver health. It is an excellent source of betaine which promotes detoxification, and also contains nitrates which have a stabilising effect on blood pressure.

Ingredients

1 large beetroot, peeled
½ a large courgette
1 apple
1 inch chunk of ginger, skin on
1 clove of garlic, peeled (optional)

Method

1. Scrub the apple and vegetables and juice all the items.

Chapter Six: Implementing Your Anti-Cancer Plan

Not Enough Time? Tips to Fit Nutrition into Your Day

The purpose of this book is to help you to change your current patterns around health and nutrition, into new habits which will serve you better. For some this can mean picking out a few new recipes and incorporating them into your week. But for others the task is just a little bit more daunting.

Have faith that once you have worked out an outline for a meal plan over a day or two, or even longer, with a bit of forward planning this can soon become effortless and automatic.

The use of kitchen gadgets can make a real time saving difference. If you are undergoing treatment and limited in your energy levels then do draw on the support of friends and loved ones by learning to ask for help.

A Stitch in Time Saves Nine

The worst time for me to think about what to eat is 5pm! That's just too late. I'm left to scavenge around in cupboards and fridges for something that can be quickly thrown together. This is the time that I'm most likely to make poor choices and it puts me under too much stress.

It is much better when I have a semblance of a weekly plan so that the ingredients for a number of meals are available. It is even better when I do some of the preparation earlier in the day. Here are some top tips for being prepared in the kitchen:

1. Evening or main meals take the most preparation so start by making a list of your favourite meals: For us this includes a roast, lentil bolognaise, sausages from the local farm, fish and something in the slow cooker (like a chicken or bean curry). That's five to begin, nearly a weeks' worth!

2. Next move on to lunches. Are you at work, out & about or at home? Stick to protein and veg in restaurants. Food on the go can be more difficult because these choices are often carb heavy. A packed lunch based on a salad may be easier - just make it the night before if you have an early start. Sometimes I do need to grab & go - so I might choose chicken kebabs with a veg & quinoa salad or a crayfish salad with some fruit.

3. Breakfast is often the easiest option and one that we are happy to repeat regularly. This makes the planning even simpler. Just have two or three options you can mix and match with.

4. You may find that it helps to allocate an hour in your week to choose one or two new recipes, and together with your favourite meals draft an outline main meal plan with ingredients for your shopping list. You can then supplement this with lunch and breakfast options, and snacks.

5. Plan a main shop (using online services if you prefer) and have an idea of where to top up shop during the week. Consider when you might need to allocate some prep time, especially if you like to include baking or other things that take time. One of my clients saves time by preparing and freezing organic vegetables into portions, which can be left in the fridge to defrost whilst he's at work.

Here's a template to help you weekly plan. You can print out fresh copies from the website. www.OutsmartCancer.co.uk

7 Day Meal Planner

W/C _____

Breakfast	Meal 1	Meal 2

OK, that's the hard bit done - you have a plan! Now on a daily basis get a little organised and you're there. This may mean taking things out of the freezer in good time, prepping in advance or using a slow cooker so that dinner is ready when you are.

Every Cook Needs Gadgets

Our grandparents would have spent a long time preparing food, but the good news is that we can really make food prep a breeze with some clever gadgets. Here are some of my favourite kitchen items which save both time and effort:

Steamer

The very best way to cook vegetables is by steaming – it preserves nutrients and is clean, easy and convenient.

As I'm microwave phobic I also use a steamer for other things such as to poach eggs, cook porridge, stew fruit and reheat soup. Mine is an electric version which means it can be switched on and then left without worry. I can pop on some eggs, for instance, and then walk the dog. It's nice to get home and find that breakfast is pretty much ready. A stove top steamer is just fine too, but this does need close supervision.

High Speed Blender

It is well worth investing in the best that you can afford, although any good quality blender, or even hand held blending stick, can get you started. High powered blenders are particularly useful for making soups in a jiffy, smoothies, sauces, nut milks, batters and spreads. The piece de resistance is the Vitamix – pricey but incredibly powerful. Alternatively, the Nutribullet is also highly recommended and is very popular for making smoothies with the minimum of fuss.

Pampered Chef Food Chopper

This is my number one gadget that even comes on holidays (self catering only!) It makes light work of chopping veg very finely to make fast and effortless salads. Not only is this more appetising but it's easier both to eat and to digest lots of vegetables if they are cut up into very small pieces. This breaks you out of thinking of salad as just lettuce and cucumber. Instead create delicious, simple salads such as red cabbage and apple with walnuts and lentils in minutes. You can also use the various blades on a food processor for this.

Food Processor

This can also be used to finely chop vegetables, and is useful if you are making a reasonable quantity. A food processor will easily blend together ingredients to make home-made burgers, falafel or meatballs. I find it easier to use for more solid foods than a blender, especially when it comes to scraping out the bowl.

I also have a mini version for making individual portions such as a quick guacamole, hummus or olive & tomato paste.

Slow Cooker

Truly a cook's best friend... and don't think about using it only in the winter. I usually put a roasting joint in at the weekend – chicken, lamb or gammon. Just add a handful of herbs as it makes its own juice. Depending on the size, it usually takes around 5 hours on a medium setting to have a delicious roast. Then, if you've bought organic, return the bones with water and any vegetable trimmings and leave overnight on a medium setting for a delicious stock.

Slow cookers are also great for cooking stews of pulses and beans, but do refer to the instructions on the packet. Some beans require pre-soaking and the instructions may suggest initially bringing them to the boil and then changing the water before simmering over time.

Juicer

Juicing is a fantastic way to dramatically increase nutrient intake. There are two main types of juicer; centrifugal juicers, which work by using a rapidly spinning sieve basket and masticating juicers which work by crushing produce using slowly rotating gears.

Masticating juicers tend to give an optimum juice yield and can maintain more nutrients than centrifugal juicers. They are more expensive and less widely available on the high street. I strongly recommend that if you are going to invest in a juicer you opt for one of these, if your budget can stretch to it.

www.UKJuicers.com offer many different models, I use an Omega Vert – a masticating juicer which is upright so it takes up less counter space.

Spiralizer

A delightful alternative to pasta – make your own spaghetti from raw courgette, carrot, mooli (also known as daikon, a Japanese radish) or other hard vegetable. I use an upright version again because of the smaller footprint. Simply spiralize the vegetables, add some dressing and a few nuts or seeds for a delicious fast food option. (These are also available from UKjuicers.com).

Bento Box

This is a posh lunch box, which is very popular with many of my clients. You may wonder how you ever existed without one! If you need to take a packed lunch then this is a great way to ensure that you have the food that you need. The Aladdin has insulation, a carry handle, is stackable so you can take multiple dishes and it looks fairly good too.

Packed lunches can also be helpful for people who work from home. When food is pre-prepared it can save time and reduce stress, particularly if you are very busy.

Sourcing Good Quality Food – Where to Buy?

I do think that sourcing food is an issue, and where possible I prefer to use local suppliers and farms, particularly those that produce their food organically.

Try to buy meat from a reputable butcher, a farm shop or, if using a supermarket, choose organic. The higher price reflects the less intensive rearing of livestock, resulting in a higher quality of meat and less contamination with antibiotics and other additives. We have very good local farm shop where the animals graze for most of the year. Their meat is delicious!

Fish is potentially more difficult to source locally, unless you live by the sea. I would be happy to hear from any fish producers who can convince me of the quality of their food. We don't have a local fish shop and so we use the supermarket. I choose wild salmon over organic as the latter is still intensively farmed. However I also use mackerel which is farmed, in moderation.

An organic box scheme is a good idea if you can't source organic produce locally. Riverford and Abel & Cole both offer national distribution in the UK and offer high quality fresh organic produce. I buy some organic products at the supermarket, and also use a local grocer. Their veg is very good but doesn't last long, which I am happy about as it suggests that they are less contaminated with chemicals to make them stay fresher for longer. Some supermarkets are now stocking less expensive produce which is not grown to their aesthetic standards, and this is worth considering if you are on a budget.

Nutrition on a Budget

When making changes towards a real food diet, cost can often be a consideration. A real food diet does cost more, however there are swings and roundabouts. Whilst you may be paying more for better quality or organic meat, and possibly for vegetables and fruits, you will be paying less for high calorie snacks and processed foods with minimal nutritional value. Many people find that there is a significant contribution to their household budget from reducing or even abstaining from alcohol.

Protein is usually the most expensive part of a dietary budget and here are some tips to make your budget go further:

- Choose cheaper cuts of meat: these are often more flavoursome and lend themselves well to slow cooking. I might choose beef shin instead of steak for a casserole, and offal like liver is incredibly nutritious and is a cheaper option than leaner cuts.

- Buy a whole chicken rather than chicken pieces. There may be meat left for a second meal or soup, and always use the bones for stock if you are able.

- Eggs are an egg-cellent choice and a frittata or quiche makes a satisfying main meal.

- Have a couple of meat free days in the week, and include pulses, nuts and seeds or goats cheese as the protein source.

- Add pulses to casseroles to add bulk and protein to a dish.

- Tinned fish such as mackerel and sardines are also economical and convenient.

Another consideration is the priority that we give to food within the household budget. When we view food as part of our healing journey, it really is worth investing as much as we can afford to spend to bring real food to the table.

As Dr Terry Wahls says in her TED talk (see Chapter Three) good food *is* more expensive, but we have the choice to either pay now or pay later. Most people aspire to maintaining a healthy and active old age, and good nutrition is a really viable way to reduce your risk of long-term ill health.

Eating Out & Pre-Prepared Food

The good news is that the *Outsmart Cancer* Plan is flexible enough to enable you to eat out quite easily, especially if you select higher quality restaurants.

Even in pizza and pasta places it is usually possible to choose wisely, either a meat or fish dish with vegetables, and/or a salad. You might even choose two starters, or ask for a small change to the menu. For example, you might ask for a side salad with soup instead of bread, or extra veg instead of potato if you are focussing on keeping your carbohydrate low.

Indian restaurants offer a lot of variety and can be particularly helpful for vegetarians as they embrace pulses, such as in a dahl. Again I would pass on the naan, and have just a small spoonful of rice along with vegetables, and a little meat or pulses. My preference is to use ghee rather than oils, so I usually ask for this.

Coffee shops can be a challenge particularly if you are avoiding dairy and/or soy. They all stock green or herbal teas though, and try not to go hungry as most of the food choices are high carb and heavy on gluten. A granola bar or small pack of dark chocolate (70% - see below) could be an occasional treat.

Although most of the time I would encourage you to prepare meals from scratch, it is helpful to know how to shop for prepared food if you need to. First of all, apply the same theory as you would do if cooking yourself – protein, vegetables, fruit, but limit the starchy carbs. It is worth reading labels.

Whereas in the past you might have focussed on calories and low fat, these are not necessarily good priorities. Instead I encourage you to look at the carbohydrate content. For example, comparing a snack of two chocolate covered rice cakes and a small bar of 70% chocolate:

	2 x chocolate rice cakes	**30g 70% chocolate**
Calories	168kcal	180kcal
Fat	8.2g	12.6g
Carbohydrate	20.8g	10.9g
Fibre	1g	3g
Net carbs	*19.8g*	*7.9g*

In the example above you can see that these two snack choices have a similar calorie content (not that it's relevant really) but the rice cakes have roughly two and a half times as much net carbohydrate as the chocolate. A very rough rule of thumb is to express carbohydrate as sugar content in teaspoons, where 1 tsp is around 5g of carbs. Hence the rice cakes are very roughly equivalent to 4 teaspoons of sugar, which runs the risk of spiking blood sugar levels with resulting sugar cravings.

So for me the chocolate (occasional treat only!) would be a better choice, less adulterated and more satisfying.

Food Preparation Techniques

The food preparation techniques that I think are worth considering are sprouting pulses, fermenting foods (probiotics), making nut milks and making bone broth. Though all of these foods can be bought readily prepared, there are advantages to being able to make your own at home.

Sprouting Pulses

This is a fabulous way to dramatically increase the nutrient content of pulses and, in the process, make them ready to eat.

You can use a simple jam jar with a muslin cloth, or invest in a tiered sprouting tray system. UKJuicers.com have a wide range available and also sell the seeds. Otherwise you can buy pulses or seeds in the supermarket (organic if possible).

Simply choose the pulses you wish to sprout - chick peas, mung beans, aduki and green lentils are a good combination. Rinse them well in water and then soak them overnight.

Drain the pulses and either spread them in the sprouting tray or tie the muslin around the jam jar neck and invert to drain completely. Water and drain twice a day and you will see the seeds begin to germinate.

After four or five days they are ready for harvest and can be added to salads, used to make bean burgers, falafel and hummus, gently stir fried or blended.

If using a tiered system you can keep the sprout supply on the go by starting on consecutive days.

Probiotic Foods

Probiotic or fermented foods are an everyday way to boost levels of good bacteria and inhibit those that are unhelpful and may contribute to poor health. These include:

1. **Yoghurt:** Natural unflavoured live yoghurt is readily available in supermarkets. You can also make your own. Yoghurt makers can easily be purchased online. If you are

avoiding cow's dairy then goats, sheep or coconut are good options.

2. **Sauerkraut:** This is a rich source of beneficial bacteria and hence extremely healthy! You can also buy it ready prepared online www.culturedprobiotics.co.uk. Unfortunately the sauerkraut in the supermarket is pasteurised, and thus does not contain live beneficial bacteria.

Alternatively, it is really easy (and cheap!) to make sauerkraut yourself, though it takes 4-7 days to brew. A recipe is below:

Ingredients

1 cabbage, 2 carrots, 2 shallots – shred in a food processor or finely chop
2 tbsp sea salt, dissolved in 125ml warm water
1 tbsp root ginger, peeled and grated
2 garlic cloves, peeled & chopped
2 tsp dill & 2 tsp fennel; or 1 tbsp juniper berries (optional)

Method

1. Place the shredded veg in a mixing bowl and add the salt water. Massage the veg gently with clean hands until liquid is released. This may take up to five or ten minutes.

2. Stir in the garlic, ginger and herbs if you choose to use these and mix well. Tightly pack the sauerkraut into a clean glass jar with a lid.

3. Continue to press firmly into the jar so that the cabbage is covered in its own juice. (Tip – place a plastic bag full of water on top to weight the cabbage below the waterline). Tightly close the lid and leave in a warm place for up to a week. Release the pressure by opening the lid and then closing on a daily basis.

4. Refrigerate after opening and use generously with salads and main meals.

3. ***Kefir:*** This is a fermented milk drink made with kefir grains – a combination of bacteria and yeasts in a matrix of protein, lipids and sugar. Traditional kefir is made at an ambient temperature overnight. Fermentation of the lactose in milk by the kefir grains produces a thin yoghurt like drink which is rich in probiotics and nutrients (vitamins A, B1, B2, B6, B12, D, folic and nicotinic acid; calcium, iron and iodine). It can be drunk on its own or added to juices and smoothies.

    If you don't fancy making your own then it can also be purchased from Riverford.co.uk.

4. ***Kombucha:*** This a fermented green tea drink and makes a lovely refreshing alternative to wine. A caution though: if your gut is unhealthy, kombucha may contribute to yeast overgrowth and so it may be better to introduce this at later stages.

For both kefir grain and kombucha starter kits see www.happykombucha.co.uk. A useful cookbook which includes fermented foods is *The Nourished Kitchen* by Jennifer McGruther.

Nut Milk

This is very worthwhile making at home. All you need is a good blender and a nut milk bag or a piece of muslin cloth.

Soak 1 cup of almonds, or other nuts, overnight. Drain and rinse then add to the blender with 1 litre of plain water. Blend at high speed and then filter through the nut milk bag or cloth. Squeeze the milk through and catch it in a clean container.

It is lovely to drink freshly made and lasts a couple of days in the fridge (shake before using if the liquid separates). Experiment too with different nuts and seeds. Sunflower and hemp milk are both really delicious!

Bone Broth

Bone broth is used all over the world by indigenous populations as a healing drink. If you have a slow cooker simply add a cooked chicken carcass and vegetable trimmings (not cruciferous veg as these can be bitter) with water and leave on a medium setting overnight or for up to 24 hours. Strain and keep in the fridge for up to 5 days.

Use it to flavour stocks and casseroles, or enjoy as a drink with some salt & pepper, and maybe ½ tsp of organic bouillon powder to tune up the flavour.

You can also use other bones from the butcher or fishmonger, and add more veg too.

Summary

This chapter aims to help you to plan and make the transition from your current eating habits to a more nutritious way of eating.

Remember that what is new and requires extra thought today will soon become a habit that you can follow with very little effort.

1. Try to make some time each week to make a rough plan of what you will eat. Pay attention to lunches, as these can be an easy meal to compromise.

2. Invest in gadgets. They save time, and make your life easier.

3. Where possible think about sourcing natural ingredients. If these are not widely available locally, could you or someone in your family consider growing some veg in the garden?

4. When you eat out just stick to the principles of protein and vegetables or salad, and be confident in asking for what you want. If buying packaged foods always check the label.

5. Experiment with some of the techniques for food preparation like sprouting, making fermented foods, nut milks and stock.

Cook from fresh when you can and prepare meals with love and gratitude. Enjoy the choices you make and, above all, be kind to yourself.

Now that you have a solid foundation for making enjoyable food choices, I am going to move on to individualising your health plan. We all have different underlying health issues and this will help you to identify where you may benefit from some added focus.

Chapter Seven: Individualising Your Programme

Do you wake up each morning feeling energised? Is your mind alert and can you easily concentrate on the task in ahead? Do you sleep well? How is your digestion? Does your skin radiate health? How high are your stress levels? Do you ever feel 'hormonal'? Is your mood balanced or do you become easily agitated or down sometimes?

Really good health isn't just about the absence of disease, it's also about living the best quality of life that our genes will allow. We should all be aiming to create a body that is as healthy as it can be, and that's why any niggley little symptoms really should be addressed.

Think of symptoms as your body's way of telling you that all is not as good as it could be. Pay attention in the early stages, and future ill health could be avoided.

If you are already in the position of having your health compromised, the same applies. Even if you have a difficult prognosis, aiming to give yourself the best health you possibly can will pay dividends. It can dictate how well you cope with treatment and could also reduce your risks of a future recurrence.

Understandably, anyone having been through a cancer experience will have some concern about whether or not their cancer will return. I was given odds of 50%, which I didn't really like very much. My GP pointed out that I just had to make sure that I was in the right 50%! So that's why I really set out on a journey of healing and recovery, not just from the cancer, but also to give myself every advantage for futureproofing my own health.

But the other really great benefit of addressing your health in totality is that you just feel so much better. Personally, my energy levels now far exceed how I felt twelve years ago (pre cancer). At the age of 39 I thought I was 'getting on a bit'; fast forward twelve years and I'm climbing mountains and cycling hundreds of miles. Over time a shopping list of niggly symptoms resolved themselves, though not without some considerable effort on my part, and I now enjoy a really active and rewarding lifestyle. With a bit of focus, you can too.

A really good diet is the cornerstone of nutritional medicine, and you may find that to take your health to the next level, supplements play an important role too. In this chapter we'll consider some key areas of potential imbalance with suggestions for how to address them. This is something you can work on yourself if you are sufficiently motivated and keen to read around the subject. Alternatively you may like to consider working with a qualified nutritionist who can guide you through the process (see Chapter Eight – finding a nutritional practitioner).

Managing Inflammation:
The Villain of Ill Health

In Chapter One you heard that inflammation is our body's way of responding to damage or injury, and that it is also one of the triggers of cancer. However inflammation is so prevalent in its association with ill health that we are going to explore it again in more detail here.

You may also be aware of the presence of inflammation where there is pain. Indeed pain relieving Non-Steroidal Anti

Inflammatory Drugs (NSAID) like ibuprofen and aspirin, and steroidal drugs like prednisolone, work by suppressing inflammation.

Although acute inflammation generally causes pain, you may also have a chronic low level of inflammation that you aren't even aware of, or that you haven't connected with the symptoms that you are experiencing. Because of the contribution of low-grade inflammation to cardiovascular and cancer risk, aspirin (which is anti-inflammatory) is often recommended as a preventative measure. However, there are also many natural products that have anti-inflammatory properties.

Inflammation is associated with many health conditions and symptoms, here are just a few:

- Weight gain and insulin resistance[154]

- Diabetes[155]

- Cancer (see Chapter One)

- Heart disease[156]

- High blood pressure[157]

- Periodontal disease[158]

- Depression[159]

- Any condition with pain, eg: arthritis, fibromyalgia

- Autoimmune conditions eg: ulcerative colitis, ankylosing spondylitis, multiple sclerosis

So in a nutshell, inflammation is more than likely going to be a factor in any symptoms or conditions that you are experiencing.

What Causes Inflammation?

The real question here is, what is causing damage internally that is resulting in an inflammatory response?

Potential causes include bacterial or viral infection, trauma, burns or the presence of toxins and other foreign materials. Basically anything that is recognised as 'foe' by the immune system, and provokes an immune response can lead to an inflammatory response. The damaged cells release chemicals which cause the blood vessels to leak fluid into the tissues, causing swelling, and attracting white blood cells to fight the infection. The resulting immune complexes continue to circulate until they are broken down or excreted as pus or mucus.

The role of gut health and potential food sensitivities deserves special mention. Your gut is home to around 100 trillion microorganisms, a number ten times greater than the total number of cells in the human body. These bacteria are vital to health because they perform a multitude of metabolic functions. An unhealthy gut may also harbour pathogenic bacteria and parasites, and these can be a source of infection.

Food sensitivities occur when particular foods are recognised as 'foe'. Wheat or gluten, dairy and soy are some of the most common. In a sensitised individual, the trigger foods cause antibodies to be produced. Full blown allergies, the reactions such as a peanut allergy which require urgent medical attention are mediated by IgE antibodies. However IgA and IgG antibodies indicate a milder sensitivity, where the impact may be insidious but can be problematic all the same.

Removing the cause of inflammation is vital to recovery. Hence you should adopt the anti-inflammatory *Outsmart Cancer* diet which is high in nutrients. You should also exclude wheat products, refined carbohydrates and sugars, all of which promote inflammation.[160] Gut health should be addressed to reduce bacterial toxicity and food sensitivity. Alongside diet, natural anti-inflammatory supplements can be employed.

Natural Anti-Inflammatories

Aloe Vera: This is a succulent plant species which is renowned for its healing properties. It can be applied topically as a gel or a cream, or the juice can be drunk. Taken internally it may reduce oxidative stress and inflammation in the digestive tract.[161] Aloe also exerts a positive effect on the growth of probiotic bacteria.[162] I have personally witnessed a client achieve a dramatic reduction in C Reactive Protein (a blood marker for inflammation) in a very short time when taking drinking aloe vera, alongside dietary improvement.

To maximise its therapeutic effect, always look for brands made from the inner gel of the whole leaf, such as Forever Living, Nutrigold or Pukka. Dosage is between 30ml and 100ml daily, on an empty stomach.

Curcumin: I talked about curcumin in Chapter One, in respect of the vast and growing volume of research around its potential anti-cancer activities. Curcumin is the active ingredient in the yellow Indian spice turmeric. Generously adding turmeric to curries and even salads can be helpful way to increase your dietary intake. Combine it with some ground black pepper to increase its bioavailability. But it really comes into its own when taken in higher concentrations as a dietary supplement.

Animal studies to support its efficacy are widely available. For instance, one study involved mice with Helicobacter pylori infection, a bacteria which is indicated as a trigger for stomach cancer. Curcumin treatment exerted a significant anti-inflammatory effect with decreased expression of inflammatory cytokines, which are immune based cell signalling molecules.[163]

In human subjects, a review of six trials concluded that curcumin demonstrates an anti-inflammatory action and is found to be safe at dosages of between 1g and up to 8g daily. This supplement was seen to inhibit a number of different molecules in the blood, all of which play a role in inflammation.[164]

Good brands to look for include Curcumin X4000, Biotics Kapparest (curcumin, boswellia, propolos, green tea, ginger, rosemary, resveratrol) or Metagenics Ultra InflamX (a protein shake with multiple nutrients, turmeric, ginger, rosemary and quercetin).

Omega 3 Fats: You may remember from Chapter Three that omega 3 fats are anti-inflammatory, and the best sources are oily fish, flax seeds and walnuts. It can also be taken as a fish oil supplement. For vegetarians or those with fish allergies, linseed oil and evening primrose oils are positive alternatives. Animal experiments and clinical intervention studies indicate that omega 3 fatty acids might be useful in a wide range of inflammatory and autoimmune diseases. Many of the placebo controlled trials reveal significant benefit to the patient, as measured by a decrease in their disease activity and a lowered need to use anti-inflammatory medications.[165]

Firstly, ensure that you have sufficient intake of omega 3 fats in relation to omega 6 fats like arachidonic acid found in animal products, which are pro-inflammatory. This ratio can be measured in a laboratory test via Genova Diagnostics (see Chapter Eight) or supplement if you have symptoms and your dietary intake is low.

Eskimo Brainsharp is a blend of omega 3 from fish and evening primrose oil, and Eskimo-3 is omega 3 only. Both are available in capsule or liquid form. If using the liquid then keep it refrigerated after opening.

Proteolytic Enzymes: These are substances that are naturally produced to break down proteins. The enzymes have the capacity to hydrolyse the peptide bonds that link amino acids together. They are vitally important as part of the process of digesting our food, but also feature systemically to remove unwanted protein and immune complexes from the blood and tissues. Hence they also have a role in the control of blood clotting, cell replication, immune response and in managing inflammation.

Taken as a supplement between meals, proteolytic enzymes contribute to breaking up circulating immune complexes, necrotic debris and excess fibrin. This can be exceptionally helpful in inflammatory conditions.[166]

Incidentally, proteolytic enzymes have a history of use as a cancer therapy. In 1902 Dr John Beard, a Professor at Edinburgh University, first proposed that trypsin, a pancreatic enzyme, might play a role against cancer. During the 1960s, his ideas were taken forwards by Dr William Kelly. Dr Gonzalez worked with Dr Kelly as an intern, and discovered that he was having remarkable success with even the most difficult cases, including pancreatic cancer, utilising enzyme therapy. Dr Gonzalez is now one of the main advocates of enzyme therapy in the world and his recent paper highlighting case reports makes fascinating reading. It is available free online.[167]

Proteolytic enzymes should be taken between meals. Do not take them with anti-coagulant medicine or with a history of gastritis or stomach ulcers.

Improving Digestive Health

How important do you think it is to have a really good digestive system?

Digestive complaints are very common, and people don't always seek medical attention. Instead they may self-medicate with laxatives, fibre or over-the-counter ant-acids. Where symptoms warrant, your GP may refer you for testing to determine if there is any underlying pathology or infection. This may include testing for a bacteria called Helicobacter pylori or for parasites, or an examination for changes in pathology to the oesophagus, small intestine or colon. Family history may suggest the need for testing for antibodies against wheat fractions which indicate gluten intolerance or even coeliac disease (this is the Cyrex test, see Chapter Eight).

Such testing may result in a diagnosis or tests may come back negative. If you still have symptoms this indicates that there may be a functional issue with the digestive system not working efficiently, as opposed to the pathological changes such as with inflammatory bowel disease (IBD), gastroesophageal reflux disease (GERD) or cancer.

Resolving digestive issues is of prime importance not just because these can be unpleasant, inconvenient or painful, but because digestion is the key process that enables you to extract the goodness and nutrients from your food. It matters little how good your food is if your digestion is sub optimal, in which case your nutrient intake will always be compromised.

A further factor which is starting to be acknowledged in the medical literature is the beneficial impact of a strong and robust bowel flora for good health. In contrast, many of us probably have fairly 'foul bowels'... I certainly did until I began on this journey of recovery and wellness. Good bacteria or probiotics are essential for good health[168]. In contrast an overgrowth of pathogenic bacteria, yeasts or parasites, will add a toxic load to our systems. Their waste products have to be processed and removed in the urine – this can be measured in an organic acid test (see Chapter Eight). Dysbiosis, which is an imbalance of microbes in the gut, can result in bacteria passing through the intestinal wall and challenging our immune system. This is not what we want when striving to outsmart cancer.

So let's take it from the top, and explore the stages of a well-functioning digestive system.

The World Within – From Food to Nutrients

Good digestion begins even before you've taken that first bite. Are you in the right frame of mind to eat, or are you expecting your digestive system to do its stuff whilst you distract yourself with something else? It is a really good practice to be in the present. If possible sit at a table and enjoy or savour each mouthful. It is even better if this is with friends or family, though that may not always practical. Chew purposefully and thoroughly. Masticate well. This breaks down particle sizes and increases the surface area on which the digestive enzymes can act. Salivary amylase in your mouth starts this process off, beginning the digestion of carbohydrates.

When you swallow your food it passes into the acidic environment of your stomach, which stores the food and churns it to further break it down. Pepsin is released which acts on protein, breaking it down into smaller molecular structures or peptides. Hydrochloric acid is secreted by specialised cells to maintain a pH of between 1 and 3 – which is very acidic. This is essential for several reasons:

- Pepsin works best in an acidic environment. Hence digestion is compromised without it.

- The acidity kills microbes ingested with your food, thus protecting you from infection.

- Nutrients such as dietary B12 are released via the action of pepsin and acid; intrinsic factor is produced in the stomach to facilitate B12's later absorption.

- The acidic chyme entering the small intestine stimulates the production of bicarbonate. This is the next stage of digestion.

The next steps occur in the duodenum and upper small intestine. Digestive enzymes and bicarbonate are released from the pancreas, and bile from the liver/ gall bladder which serves to emulsify and break down fats. These digestive juices continue to break down large molecules into tiny units of amino acids (from protein), glycerol and fatty acids (from fats) and di-saccharides (from carbohydrates). At the same time, bile discharges waste products including hormones, toxic metabolites and cholesterol from the liver into the intestinal tract for removal via the faeces.

Further down in the small intestine more enzymes are produced. These break down the disaccharides into individual monosaccharides, mainly glucose. Here the fully broken down fats, proteins and carbs are absorbed, as well as the vitamins, minerals, polyphenols and other phytonutrients that were in your foods.

The large intestine or colon reduces the loss of water, salts and nutrients by reabsorbing these, which ultimately forms the stool. The majority of bacterial action takes place in the colon.

Stool evacuation should be regular, at least once a day and twice or even three times is perfectly normal with a good diet. The stool should be easy to pass, of a soft but firm consistency and, although not pleasant, should not be foul smelling. Constipation risks the recirculation of toxicity which is not efficiently removed from the body. On the other hand urgency or diarrhoea, loose stools or going consistently more than 3 times daily may indicate that the body is trying to rid itself of something. Food sensitivities should be considered.

Leaky Gut and Food Sensitivities

A consequence of digestive distress is that the cells of the intestinal lining may become increasingly irritated, causing inflammation. Leaky gut syndrome arises when the integrity of the gut wall is challenged, and there is a breakdown of the molecules which are responsible for maintaining the tight junctions between the epithelial cells. The role of these cells is to allow nutrients to pass through to the bloodstream whilst keeping microbes, toxins, waste products and undigested food out. However, once the barrier has become compromised, undesirable molecules are able to pass freely into the bloodstream, provoking an immune response and increasing inflammation as described earlier in this chapter. Such a leaky gut can set the stage for autoimmune diseases[169] or for illnesses which thrive when there is a weakened immune system, as in cancer.[170]

As described earlier, food allergies arise when the immune system recognises particular foods as foe, and makes antibodies to attack them. You should also consider the possibility of food sensitivities. These relate to foods that trigger a reaction from your white blood cells. They may not raise an immune response, and for this reasons are often referred to as "masked food allergies". They too can cause devastating symptoms.

Food intolerance testing can be considered as part of a digestive health programme; this assesses the presence of antibodies to specific food proteins in the blood. After avoidance of the offending foods, the ultimate the goal is to 'heal and seal' the gut so that intestinal integrity is re-established.

It may be appropriate to assess intestinal permeability. This, along with auto-immunity and reactivity to wheat, can be measured via a Cyrex profile (see Chapter Eight).

Restoring Gut Health Naturally

You can see now how important it is to have good digestion. This will give you a maximum intake of nutrients in combination with the efficient removal of waste products from your system.

So what do you do when all is not well with your digestion? This is when a 4 stage 4R programme is beneficial: Remove, Replace, Reinoculate and Repair.

1. **Remove:** First off all, clean up your diet. If you need yet another reason for eliminating refined carbohydrates, then here it is. Sugar feeds pathogenic bacteria and yeasts in your gut. The sugars are fermented for an energy supply, releasing gases which may contribute to windiness and bloating.

    Secondly, remove foods to which you are sensitive. A good start point is to eliminate wheat, dairy and soy as these are the top allergenic foods. If your digestion is very bad you may want to go so far as removing all grains and possibly even legumes or pulses. This is the Paleo version of the *Outsmart* eating plan. Paleo eating is gaining a strong following amongst people with digestive problems.

Finally, anti-microbials can be used to remove pathogenic bacteria, yeasts or parasites. If you are seeing a Nutritional Practitioner they may suggest a stool test so that a specific anti-microbial programme can be determined and established. This is not essential, but it can help to inform a specific treatment plan and is thus one that is more individualised to you.

I often recommend **Designs for Health GI-Microb-X** which is a blend of natural extracts with a long history of use as antimicrobials including caprylic acid, uva ursi, grapefruit seed extract, wormwood, black walnut and berberine. Nutri offer an effective botanical blend called Berberine & Grapefruit seed. Oil of oregano, such as Biotics ADP, can be used alongside a broad spectrum anti-microbial, or on its own, particularly when a yeast overgrowth is suspected or determined via testing.

The active ingredient of garlic, allicin, also has antimicrobial properties[171] and so regularly including garlic within your diet will confer some protective advantage.

Acid reflux is a common condition in people eating Westernised diets, and many are prescribed medication either taking an over the counter remedy or prescription drugs. Where there is stomach pain or reflux (dyspepsia), mastic gum can offer natural relief and be used alongside ant-acid medication like lansoprazole or omeprazole. Mastica is a traditional natural remedy used throughout the Eastern Mediterranean. Taken as a supplement, it has been shown to significantly reduce dyspepsia in a patient group compared to placebo.[172] Extracts of mastic gum are effective against Helicobacter Pylori infection, which is a cause of stomach ulcers and a risk factor for stomach cancer.[173]

2. ***Replace:*** Efficient digestion requires a plentiful supply of digestive juices. Firstly ensure a sufficient production of stomach acid as this initiates protein digestion. Excessive burping may indicate insufficiency. In this case HCl tablets taken with meals help to acidify your stomach contents. The use of apple cider vinegar either in salad dressings or taken in water before meals can also aid digestion.

   As we age and in acute and chronic illness, our digestive capacity can be compromised. Stomach and pancreatic enzymes taken at the end of meals, either with or without HCl, can support digestive function. Bile salts are essential for fat digestion.

Nutri Nutrigest is a combined product containing HCl, pancreatic enzymes and ox bile. A vegetarian option is Nutri's Similase, or BioNutri's Ecogest, which also contains probiotics.

High levels of fat in the stool, indicated either from a stool test or if the stool appears 'greasy' and floats, suggests that bile production is insufficient. Constipation may also indicate a deficiency of bile. The use of bile extracts such as Biotics Beta Plus or Nutri Gall Plus can be a useful addition, particularly if you have had gall bladder surgery. However in order to stimulate bile production you must be eating good fats in your diet.

3. ***Reinoculate:*** The importance of a healthy gut flora was discussed in Chapter Two in relation to outsmarting cancer.

   Probiotic supplements can be helpful when there are low levels of health giving microbes including acidophilus and bifidobacterium in the gut. This may be indicated by symptoms such as stomach pain, bloating, constipation or diarrhoea which often improve with supplementation.[174] A course of antibiotics will deplete good bacteria, and natural antibiotics may have a similar effect. Again, stool testing can pinpoint levels of the good bacteria present in an individual and this can assist in determining probiotic dosage. It is helpful but not essential.

There are many good brands of probiotic on the market, for example from Nutri, Nutrigold and Biocare. Look for potency between 15 billion organisms to 120 billion organisms, but in most cases start slowly and build up to ensure tolerability. In people who are particularly sensitive, or with children, Biokult is a broad spectrum probiotic containing 14 different strains and has a potency of 2 billion organisms per capsule. I often recommend the brand Culturelle for patients who are being treated with chemotherapy. It contains Lactobacillus GG, a probiotic which has been rigorously tested and researched, including alongside chemotherapy.[175]

Alongside an antimicrobial programme, I may recommend Saccharomyces Boulardii, a probiotic yeast. This can be taken with antibiotics and used in combination with regular probiotics.

Whilst probiotics play a useful role in re-establishing a healthy gut flora, do not underestimate the power of fermented foods as a source of natural probiotics. These include kefir, kombucha, live yoghurt and sauerkraut which are discussed in Chapter Six.

4. **Repair:** The final stage of the 4R gut restoration programme is to optimise the health of the epithelial cells lining the digestive tract.

Glutamine, an amino acid derived from protein, has been shown in many studies to improve intestinal barrier function. For example in a recent randomised control study with children in Brazil, glutamine supplementation resulted in a significant reduction in intestinal permeability.[176] Glutamine is best supplemented away from meals, at a suggested dosage of 5g daily (1tsp) dissolved in water. A good time to take this is before bed. A useful combination product is Nutri Glutagenics, which contains glutamine, aloe vera and liquorice to support the intestinal health.

Other options include bovine colostrum, which has a beneficial effect in preventing small intestine injuries from painkiller administration in rats.[177] Those supplemented with colostrum had less intestinal permeability, reduced bacterial overgrowth and less damage to the mucosal villi. A recommended brand is Biotics Research Immuno gG.

Butyric acid (Biocare) and N acetyl glucosamine (Nutri Permeability Factors) may also be considered. In addition, zinc, vitamin A and vitamin D have a role to play in the maintenance of gut health.

Unleash the Power of Your Mind

Stress affects people in different ways. Some people, when faced with challenges, seem to sail on without a care in the world, yet for others even the slightest thing can cause anxiety and distress. Even the same situation can be perceived very differently by two different individuals. Some people thrive on stress, whilst for others it can be completely debilitating.

Stress can initiate our 'fight or flight' response, and is designed to keep us safe and remove us from danger. When we sense a threat in our environment, whether real or imagined, powerful hormones are triggered which flood through our bloodstream and cause physiological changes. In a nano second our body is primed for action; heart rate and blood pressure is increased to deliver more oxygen, blood is diverted to the major muscle groups, digestion is slowed and blood glucose levels are boosted. It can make us more focussed and our sense of pain may be diminished.

The two hormones responsible for the stress response are adrenaline and cortisol. Both are produced in the adrenal glands which sit above the kidneys, and so are referred to as 'adrenal hormones'.

This emergency system serves us well as an acute response. However, life in the 21st century is largely safe from external or acute dangers. Many of us though experience chronic and ongoing low grade stress which can, over time, wreak havoc on our health.

Diagnosis of a serious health condition like cancer will put most people into a tail spin to a greater or lesser extent. There can be elements of fear about what the future may bring. Worry about the effect on our families. Anger at why it happened to us, and a whole range of other emotions capable of exerting stress on our system. These feelings are real and shouldn't be denied or suppressed, but for the sake of our health and recovery we need to find a way to manage those feelings and minimise their negative effects.

The Effects of Chronic Stress

The Autonomic Nervous System (ANS), which controls involuntary actions such as breathing, the beating of your heart, digestion and other necessary bodily functions, is comprised of two main sub-systems: the sympathetic and parasympathetic nervous systems.

The sympathetic nervous system is responsible for the 'flight or fight' response, which we have been discussing. Through the release of the powerful hormones adrenaline and cortisol we are able to 'power up' and deal with our stressors in a physical sense.

The parasympathetic nervous system can be referred to as 'rest and digest', and this controls general body maintenance.

The issue with spending too much time in a 'fight or flight' state is that there is a down regulation of the 'rest & digest' state. As an analogy consider when you have an important task to finish. You are unlikely to spend time on more mundane and less urgent activities like, for instance, mopping the kitchen floor. In the same way your body will prioritise the stress response over general housekeeping and maintenance of bodily functions. No point in digesting your food if you are about to be eaten by a tiger – far better to give you the resources to run away…. fast. And the thing is, the stress response is exactly the same whether you are in danger of attack, anxious at your work or concerned about your health.

Furthermore, constantly elevated levels of the stress hormone cortisol can lead to the suppression of your immune system which is, in the longer term, undesirable. Stress can accelerate DNA damage, which has implications for cancer.[178] Stress-prone personalities and negative emotional responses are related to higher cancer incidence and poorer cancer survival.[179]

Should You Just Put on a Brave Face?

To really feel the healing benefits of reducing stress it is not enough just to pretend, to yourself or others, that you are absolutely fine. Your body doesn't lie, and even if the feelings are suppressed they will still be physiologically active.

But there are things that you can do to gain a better perspective on your situation, to bring hope and peace, laughter and friendship, and relaxation into your world.

Strategies for Managing Stress

Talking Therapies

Counselling gives you the opportunity to work through your thoughts and feelings in order to make sense of them. Your GP may be able to refer you for counselling support, or you may choose to see someone privately. There are two cancer charities with help lines that you can call for support – Yes to Life and the Penny Brohn Cancer Care Centre (see Resources). You may be in touch with a cancer buddy going through treatment at the same time as you, or you may have links to a local cancer support group. Perhaps you have a friend who is good at listening. For those of you linked to a local place of worship, there is tremendous power in prayer and your church, synagogue or mosque may also offer some pastoral support.

Meditation & Visualisation

Take the time just to sit and be still. Meditation is a state of deep concentration. It brings the mind to a focus and cuts out the 'mental chatter' that we tend to carry around with us.

Visualisation is a type of meditation where the focus involves a mental image. You create in your mind the experience of doing something in great detail, and this can have an impact on both your thoughts and your body by reducing stress levels.

In my recovery I consistently visualised my daughter's wedding day. I could see her, smell her, and imagine her hair, the detail of her dress, the flowers. She was only 6 at the time but imagining her as a grown up gave me a real sense of being part of her future. It gave me a tranquil place to go when the going got tough. It also became part of my day just to get my thoughts in the right place.

There are lots of resources for guided meditations and visualisations on the internet. www.InMindInBody.com offer a visualisation wellness club specifically to help you optimise your health or improve recovery from illness. You are guided through the visualisation which can be a useful way of engaging your mind in a positive and reflective way. Interestingly, research shows that this doesn't just facilitate healing, but can also contribute to real physiological change.[180]

Love to Laugh

When did you last laugh out loud? Children do it all the time, but as adults it may be quite a rarity. Yet laughter floods you with good feelings and joy, and it's impossible to be angry or sad or anxious when you smile. The good news is that your brain can't tell whether your laughter is fake or real, and so just the act of making yourself laugh can be beneficial.

In addition, laughter boosts endorphins (your feel good hormones), reduces cortisol and adrenaline and boosts the T lymphocytes of your immune system – so it is the perfect stress-buster!

When we run *Outsmart Cancer* workshops we always try to include a Laughter Yoga session for this reason. It is quite astonishing how the energy in the room can change from such a simple act. Again, there are lots of videos on the internet for you to find out more, and there may even be a laughter club local to you. One of my favourite resources is www.robertrivest.com.

Of course, if that doesn't appeal to you, try watching a funny film, hanging out with friends who make you laugh, or taking in some comedy shows.

Exercise

Exercise is very beneficial for lots of reasons. It is motivating and stimulating (brain health). It builds muscle (including the heart), strengthens bones and ligaments, encourages deeper breathing (promoting lung health) and energises us.

Exercise can also help reduce stress levels by increasing feel good endorphins, improve sleep and mood, or help you shed worries and anxiety by focussing on something different.

When you are well, finding a sport or activity that you love to do can give you extra motivation and get-up-and-go. A balanced exercise routine should include three elements:

- Cardio – builds stamina - walking, cycling, swimming

- Resistance – builds strength – gym work, weights

- Flexibility – yoga, pilates, etc.

On the other hand, if you are going through treatment or unable to exercise, just try to get outside for fresh air when you can. Even a simple short walk can raise your spirits. Failing that, take the time to visualise an activity you love, and at least gain some benefit from imagining what it would feel like.

Energy Therapies – Reiki, Reflexology, Acupuncture, Healing etc.

One of the most profound experiences I had was to work with a spiritual healer. As often happens if you believe in Karma at all, this healer was introduced to us locally at just the time of my diagnosis. I had weekly sessions which involved an alleged transfer of energy. Sounds whacky, I know, but you really had to be there! My husband, Andy, is very sceptical about things like this but, quite frankly, he was amazed. The healer stood behind me and could move my body, without touching me. Andy said his hands glowed, and called him the Ready Brek man! I always felt better afterwards. So whatever it was doing was worth it. Just having a session of focussing your mind on healing can only be a good thing.

The other service that was available through the oncology department was reflexology, and this I found very beneficial too. If you are going through treatment, then find out what services your hospital may offer. And if you're in the realms of prevention, consider any treatments which restore energy flow and enhance well-being. They can all be a very good investment in your health and your future.

Supplements

There are a number of supplements which may help to promote a more relaxed state. BioNutri Neuralactin contains magnesium, B vitamins and theanine which can be helpful when anxiety is affecting sleep. Nutri Adreset is a blend of rhodiola, ginseng and cordyceps which provides support for those who are feeling drained and exhausted.

Boosting Your Metabolism and Energy

Low energy levels make everything seem hard, difficult and too much trouble. Fatigue is one of the main issues that people seek out a Nutritional Therapist.

There is no one organ in the human body that is responsible for making energy. Rather, each and every cell within you has the capacity to make its own energy, and this takes place in tiny organelles called mitochondria.

As the powerhouse of the cell, the mitochondria act like mini batteries, using oxygen to release the energy from our food. A pathway known as the citric acid cycle makes the necessary steps to convert glucose into Adenosine Tri Phosphate (ATP) which is the currency of your energy supply.

The efficient production of cellular energy, which results in you feeling energised, is dependent on having a steady supply of glucose, or Acetyl Co A which is the molecule derived either from glucose or fatty acids. It also requires lots of nutrients to make the necessary conversions, and an absence of toxins or heavy metals which may interfere with energy production.

In contrast, smaller amounts of energy can also be produced by glycolysis or fermentation, and this takes place in the cytosol, or gel like substance within the cell and surrounding the various organelles. You may remember that this is the preferred energy source of cancer cells. It is also a backup pathway for regular cells when their aerobic capacity is exceeded. Glycolysis doesn't require oxygen, and results in the production of lactic acid - you may be familiar with the muscle ache associated with lactic acid build up after periods of intensive exertion.

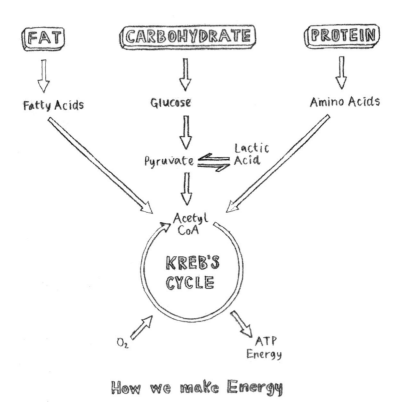

How we make Energy

Fig 5: Kreb's cycle

Back to Blood Sugar and Low Glycaemic Carbs

A steady supply of glucose and/ or fatty acids is necessary for energy production. When resources are scarce, you can also make glucose from protein in your liver, a process called gluconeogenesis, and this happens when your body breaks down muscle. Ensuring that you have regular meal times should help you to maintain, and maybe even improve, your muscle mass.

Carbohydrates are the main source of energy, and the focus is on Low Glycaemic (GL) carbs which break down slowly and provide a steady stream of glucose. These are provided by lots of colourful vegetables, and controlled portions of the more starchy carbs (root veg, some grains such as oats and rice, and fruit).

Processed, refined and excessive starchy carbs (high GL) cause a sugar rush, ie: a rapid increase in the amount of glucose in the blood. However, vital though glucose is, you can have too much of a good thing. When blood glucose runs too high, which happens in a diabetic state, it can be very damaging to peripheral blood vessels, the eyes and kidneys. Hence your body will quickly act to protect you by releasing insulin, the blood sugar regulation hormone produced in the pancreas.

Where Does Excess Sugar Go?

Initially, insulin helps the glucose molecules to enter the cells where they are utilised for energy production. But over time and in cases of continued excess, the cells may become resistant to insulin, and this could mark the start of a progression towards diabetes. In this case, the excessive sugar is escorted to the liver where it is converted into fat, which then sits around your middle. A 'muffin top' is indicative of excessive refined or starchy carb intake, courtesy of insulin. A body composition analysis may also confirm high levels of visceral fat, which sits around the organs and increases cardiovascular risk.

But from an energy point of view this surge of sugar is also bad news. Instead of being available to your cells to make energy, you can end up wearing your energy resources around your middle and your cells are denied and hungry. This drives cravings, often for the high carb and sweet foods, which perpetuate the problem. Yet despite the high calorie intake, you are likely to feel tired and low in energy.

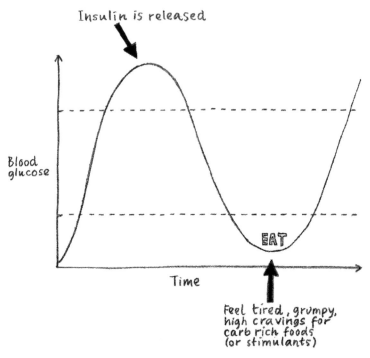

Insulin is released

Blood glucose

EAT

Time

Feel tired, grumpy, high cravings for carb rich foods (or stimulants)

The Blood Sugar Rollercoaster – refined carbohydrates lead to rapid swings in blood sugar levels.

The way out of this vicious cycle is to focus on the foods listed in the eating plan in Chapter Four. High quality, unprocessed natural foods will provide you with a steady flow of blood sugar, which your cells can utilise to make energy efficiently.

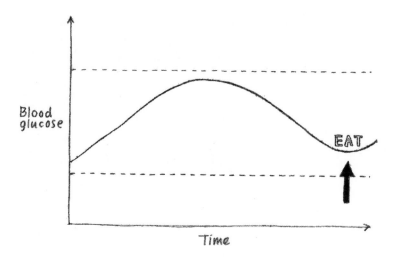

Keeping you fuller for longer—
Complex carbohydrates are more sustaining

What About Nutrients?

Many nutrients are required to convert glucose and fatty acids into energy. Some of the steps require amino acids, which come from the protein that you eat. B vitamins and magnesium are also essential. Chromium makes a complex with insulin to facilitate the movement of glucose into the cell.

Co enzyme Q10 is a supplement I took in recovery and felt amazing benefits from in terms of energy. CoQ10 is a fat soluble nutrient which has an antioxidant function and helps to protect the mitochondria against damage. It plays a unique role in some of the biochemical transformations that take place to produce energy. CoQ10 is made in the liver, but in times of ill health you may not produce it in sufficient quantities. It is important to know that statin medication, which is prescribed to lower cholesterol in the blood, interferes with the same enzyme that produces CoQ10. Hence supplementation should be considered in particular alongside medication.

Nutrients to maintain flexibility of cell membranes are also essential to ensure the ease of movement of molecules into and out of the cell. The cell membrane is a lipid-lipid bi-layer and having the right type of fats available will contribute to its own health. In particular the omega 3 fats from flax seeds and fish oils are required.

There is a very good test available which can assess any blocks in the production of energy via the citric acid cycle. In the same way that a car mechanic may assess exhaust emissions to determine how well a car engine is functioning, the organic acid test (Chapter Eight) analyses metabolites in the urine. This can highlight specific nutritional needs for that individual, and enable a focussed nutritional programme.

What Else Do I Need to Know?

Free radicals are all around us, in the air that we breathe and produced by our own metabolism. They cause the oxidative stress we discussed in Chapter One, and antioxidants protect us from their ravages. Sometimes energy production can be impaired because free radicals have damaged cell membranes, including those of the mitochondria themselves.

A high nutrient diet helps to protect you from oxidative stress, but there are times when additional support may be beneficial. Two particular times may be when you are taking very heavy exercise – where there is an increase in the volume of free radicals produced - or when you are exposed to increased oxidative stress including chemotherapy or radiation therapy.

Some oncologists are reticent about encouraging supplements alongside cancer treatment, fearing that the treatments may be affected. Yet a study of 4,877 women with breast cancer showed that the use of antioxidant supplements alongside chemotherapy was associated with an 18% reduced mortality risk and 22% reduced recurrence risk.[181] The other significant benefit of using supplements alongside cancer treatment is a reduction in side effects. One of my favourites is Propax Gold, which has the advantage of a number of clinical trials supporting its use. It is a high quality multivitamin with CoQ10 and fish oil, but with a proprietary ingredient known as NT factor which is believed to help repair cell membranes. When used alongside chemo, a reduction in adverse effects was reported in 57 – 70% of patients.[182] One of the most significant benefits is in helping to improve energy levels.

Achieving Hormonal Balance

Hormones are chemical messengers which instruct your cells in what to do. They regulate a whole host of physiological activities, including digestion, metabolism, sleep, reproduction, growth, lactation, stress and mood. Produced in glands, hormones are released into the blood stream and circulate until they reach their target cells. Here they bind to specific receptor proteins and can influence actions performed by that cell. They are incredibly powerful and generally only a small amount is required to alter cell metabolism.

For the purposes of this section, we are going to focus only on the sex hormone oestrogen.

Oestrogen

Oestrogens are the primary female sex hormones responsible for the reproductive cycle. Like other steroid hormones, they are derived from cholesterol and produced primarily by the ovaries and, during pregnancy, by the placenta. Smaller amounts are produced in the adrenal glands, liver, breasts and fat cells. The adrenals are an important source of oestrogens in post-menopausal women.

There are three naturally occurring oestrogens – estrone (E1), estradiol (E2) and estriol (E3). Estrone (E1) is found in higher concentrations after the menopause. Estradiol (E2) is the most potent, and dominant in premenopausal women. Estriol (E3) is the weakest, and this is predominant during pregnancy.

The link with oestrogen and cancer risk arises because this is a hormone which encourages proliferation of the cells in the uterus and breast tissue. More general symptoms of hormonal imbalance in women include pre-menstrual tension, mood swings, painful breasts, painful periods and heavy flow. Addressing potential imbalances early on may be an effective risk reduction strategy for cancer.

Oestrogens are repeatedly broken down in your body and excreted, and knowledge of these metabolic pathways can be helpful in understanding cancer risk. Breakdown of oestrogen takes place in a two-step process.

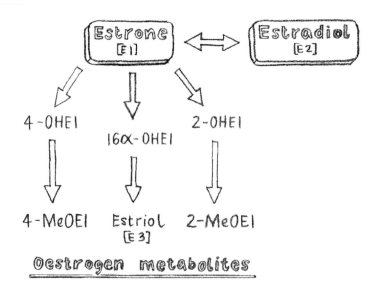

Oestrogen metabolites

In Phase 1, estrone is oxidised and there are three possible outcomes depending on which particular enzyme is involved. Elevated levels of 4-hydroxy and 16-alpha-hydroxy estrone, may be associated with higher rates of breast cancer. However 2-

hydroxyestrone is regarded as protective and higher levels generally reflect favourable oestrogen metabolism, in terms of breast health. Hence the relative amounts of these first stage metabolites can affect cancer risk.

The phase 2 step requires methylation, which involves the addition of a methyl group (carbon with three hydrogen atoms) to render the metabolites harmless before excretion.[183]

Dietary intervention can help to manipulate these metabolic pathways. Such intervention includes:

1. **Promoting a Healthy Ratio of Phase 1 Metabolites:**

- Increase cruciferous vegetables (broccoli, kale etc) and/or supplement with diindolylmethane (DIM) or indole-3-carbinol (I-3-C).[184]
- Increase your intake of berries[185] and flax seeds.[186]
- Reduce sugar consumption[187], omega 6 fats and pesticides.[188]

2. **Supporting Healthy Methylation:**

- Ensure sufficient vitamin B12, folate and sulphur containing amino acids (methionine and cysteine from meat, onions and garlic).

The good news is that these recommendations are completely consistent with the *Outsmart Cancer* diet, which is based on plentiful wholefoods. For supplements consider Nutri Meta I3C or DIM 100mg. Nutri Methyl Complex provides B12 and folate.

Summary

Addressing underlying symptoms is a powerful way both to reduce your risk of future illness, and to assist your recovery. In Chapter Two we explored the role of supporting detoxification and immune health, which applies to anyone who is concerned about cancer or simply wishing to adopt a healthy lifestyle.

In this chapter, we have explored some of the main individual considerations which may, or may not, apply to you. An overall knowledge of these potential elements will put you in a stronger position to chart your own journey back to optimal health. This can be done as a staged process, so don't feel overwhelmed if you can identify with many of the areas for improvement.

In this section I have discussed:

1. ***Inflammation:*** Supplements that can help including aloe vera, curcumin, omega 3 fats and enzymes.

2. ***Improving digestive health:*** A 4R program for restoring good gut health.

3. ***Managing stress:*** How the power of your mind can be harnessed to promote wellbeing.

4. ***Boosting your energy & metabolism:*** Low glycaemic foods help to sustain energy production.

5. ***The metabolic pathways of oestrogen:*** The importance of low sugar and a high cruciferous vegetable intake.

The final chapter in *Outsmart Cancer* considers some of the clinical tests that are available to give you some insight into underlying health imbalances. They, and the results you get, can underpin the strategies discussed in Chapter Seven.

Additional testing may not be for everyone, but I want to include it to give you a sense of what is available and how it may be relevant.

Chapter Eight:
The Health Detective

Here I describe a number of clinical tests that can be very useful either in early detection alongside conventional screening, to support you during treatment, or to help restore you to optimal health following successful medical treatment.

With the exception of conventional blood tests, which are routinely run in the health service, these tests are available privately via a Qualified Nutritionist, Naturopath, or an Integrative Doctor. The tests differ from those run by your GP in that they are exploring how well your body is functioning (hence the term Functional Medicine) rather than its pathology (where there is a definable change in tissue or organ structure). This has the advantage of enabling you to focus on improving health through supporting areas of imbalance.

Some private health policies will cover the cost of testing, but may not always include the consultation costs of your practitioner.

Your practitioner will determine the right profile of tests for you after taking a full case history. All of the tests are described on my website www.InspiredNutrition.co.uk and many of them have files attached which discuss the tests in greater detail.

Conventional Blood Tests

Whilst your doctor takes responsibility for interpreting your blood tests, requesting a copy of the test results can be very informative. Your results are compared to a normal population, known as the reference range. Here is an outline of each of the main markers in order to give you just a brief overview of what they may indicate.

Haematology

Red blood cells – are responsible for transporting oxygen around your body. Measures include red cell count, haemoglobin (the oxygen carrying molecule), the size of an average red blood cell (MCV), the width (RDW), the average weight of haemoglobin present (MCH) and the average haemoglobin concentration (MCHC).

Insufficiency of haemoglobin, or anaemia, lowers the oxygenation of the blood and may be associated with weakness, fatigue and/or shortness of breath. Common causes are blood loss (such as trauma or gastrointestinal bleed), decreased cell production (iron, B12, B6 or folate deficiency) or increased cell breakdown (due to infection, autoimmune disease or a genetic condition eg: sickle cell anaemia).

White blood cells – are the cells of the immune system which respond to infection and inflammation. The different types on a standard blood profile include *neutrophils* (defend against bacterial or fungal infection), *lymphocytes* (more common in the lymphatic system than the blood, they make antibodies to bind to pathogens), *eosinophils* (primarily deal with parasitic infections, and are the predominant cells in allergic reactions), *basophils* (release histamine to dilate blood vessels in an allergic response) and *monocytes* (dual role to present pathogens to the lymphocytes and remove cell debris).

High levels of white blood cells may be associated with an acute infection, whereas low levels indicate a more chronic picture.

When going through chemotherapy, white blood cell counts dramatically fall and are at their lowest point 7-14 days following treatment. This is why you are at a heightened risk of developing infections when undergoing chemotherapy.

Electrolytes & Kidney Function

Sodium & potassium - potassium is the most abundant mineral inside of the cells, whereas sodium is predominant in the extra-cellular fluid. Levels are controlled by kidney function and may be affected by dehydration and diuretic medication. Abnormal levels of potassium and sodium may indicate kidney disease or disturbed adrenal function – either low (hypo) or high (hyper).

Creatinine – is produced primarily by muscles when they contract, and is removed by the kidneys. It is a useful marker for kidney function. Congestion in the urinary tract can cause a back-up into the kidneys and impact normal renal function. Hence high levels may indicate inflammation or infection such as in benign prostate hypertrophy (BPH), prostatitis or a urinary tract infection (UTI). Low levels may indicate low muscle tone or a sedentary lifestyle.

Urea – is the final product of protein metabolism. It is removed via the kidneys and hence gives information on renal function, however a significant amount may also be produced in cases of gut bacterial overgrowth (dysbiosis). Bacteria acting on protein substrates generate ammonia, which is converted to urea in the liver.

Liver Function

Alkaline phosphatase, AST, ALT and GGT - these are liver enzymes. High levels may indicate an obstruction in the biliary system (from the gall bladder), damage to liver cells or liver dysfunction. Raised ALT may occur in fatty liver disease. AST also occurs in heart muscle and very high levels could be indicative of cardiovascular dysfunction.

Low levels of alkaline phosphatase may indicate low zinc status. High GGT or low AST/ ALT may suggest B6 insufficiency or high alcohol intake. GGT may also be raised with pancreatic insufficiency or pancreatitis.

Bilirubin – is formed from the breakdown of haemoglobin (known as haemolysis); it is processed in the liver and excreted in the bile. If levels are raised there may be an issue either with increased haemolysis, or a downstream problem with excretion involving liver/ biliary function

Metabolic

Cholesterol, HDL, LDL: when enquiring about your cholesterol levels, always check your HDL (otherwise known as 'good' cholesterol) reading. HDL should be at least 20% of your total cholesterol level. High cholesterol, particularly LDL (or 'bad' cholesterol), can be associated either with increased oxidative stress and/or a diet high in carbohydrates. If your diet is good and your cholesterol is high, consider asking your practitioner to test for Apolipoprotein A & B privately. Recent research is showing an association between low levels of Apo A-1 and risk of heart disease and cancer.[189]

Triglycerides - high triglycerides may be indicative of a diet too high in carbohydrate, and is associated with an increased risk of insulin resistance and cardiovascular disease.

Glucose: fasting blood glucose will highlight the risk of diabetes, and is often the consequence of a diet too high in carbohydrates. HbA1C is a longer term marker, which assesses the degree to which red blood cells are glycosylated (otherwise known as 'sugar coated').

Early Detection

Breast Thermography

Breast thermography uses a specialised infra-red camera to detect temperature increases within breast tissue.

Malignant tumour cells have an increased rate of growth compared to regular cells. Their active cell division calls for accelerated metabolism and is supported by increased blood flow. This results in an increased temperature in the tumour cells and in surrounding tissue. [190]

Thermography is a test of physiology, yielding information about the activity of cells within the breast and, like mammography, can only indicate the possibility of the presence of cancer and other breast conditions. A biopsy is always needed to confirm a diagnosis of cancer.

Thermography acts as a potential early warning of abnormal physiology. In one study of women reported to have false positive thermograms (ie: positive thermogram and negative mammogram), over one third went on to have confirmed breast cancer within five years.[191]

The benefit of such early detection, sometimes before a tumour is large enough to be confirmed by conventional means, results either in earlier treatment, or a window of opportunity.

It is recommended that a positive thermogram is followed up with conventional investigations (mammography, biopsy), to establish whether or not a tumour is present. If positive, then cancer therapy can be initiated sooner rather than later and this is of particular consequence for fast growing tumours. However, a false positive enables dietary and lifestyle intervention aimed at correcting the environment which facilitates the survival of cancer cells and enables them to thrive. Clinical testing looking at bloodwork, vitamin D status, iodine status and oestrogen metabolism may be considered.

Thermography is not a substitute for routine mammograms. Rather it is recommended in addition to regular screening and has the potential either for earlier intervention or true preventative medicine.

Cost: £200 - £300

The CA Profile

Dr Xandria Williams PhD is an authority on a range of blood tests designed to indicate the very earliest possible sign of cancer cell activity. Her belief, which has been described in this book, is that cancer is a *process* of cellular change that leads, over a long period of time, to the formation of a tumour. The sooner you detect the beginning of this process, the sooner you can take active nutritional and lifestyle steps to restore health and well-being. Like the use of early thermograms, we are considering the prevention of a cancer situation.

A range of tests are described in Dr Williams' book, Detecting Cancer.[192] One of these is the CA1 profile from American Metabolic Laboratories. The profile is composed of eight tests:

Three variants of HCG – human chorionic gonadotrophin: this hormone is associated with pregnancy (at higher levels than measured here), and is also commonly elevated in malignancy.

PHI - an enzyme which is up regulated in cancer and suggests that increasing anaerobic activity is taking place in the cytosol (aerobic respiration of healthy cells takes place in the mitochondria). A raised level of **PHI** can also encourage the development of cancer cells.

CEA - levels should be low in a healthy person, and high levels may indicate the presence of cancer.

TSH or thyroid stimulating hormone – acts on the thyroid gland to stimulate the release of thyroxine. Many of those who are developing cancer have elevated TSH, indicating a potential hypothyroid condition (low thyroxine) which results in a lowered metabolic rate. A raised TSH indicates that the body is trying to step up thyroxine production.

GGT – this has already been mentioned in the context of the conventional blood test and is a sensitive enzyme for monitoring the liver and bile system. The liver is the prime detoxification organ and often has abnormal function in malignancies, resulting in raised levels.

DHEA - the anti-stress and longevity hormone. This can indicate adrenal fatigue and many cancer patients and those developing cancer have low levels.

The CA profile is especially relevant to those post cancer, who are wishing to be diligent about monitoring future risk.

Cost: c. £300

Functional & Nutritional Tests

Functional testing offers a more subtle look at your wonderful world within, and helps to determine sub-optimal biochemical pathways or nutritional deficiencies that, if left unchecked, could contribute to the creation of a disease state.

Vitamin D

This can either be run by your GP or ordered as a home test for around £30. You simply provide a blood spot and send it to the lab in the mail.

I recommend that all cancer patients take a Vitamin D test as it is impossible to guess who may be deficient, though most are. One of my clients lives in very sunny climes, yet his Vitamin D was rock bottom.

Optimal levels are 100-200 nmol/L (40-80ng/ml). Robust Vitamin D is important for immune health, however it can be toxic at very high levels (hence the importance of testing before supplementation).

Organic Acid Test

The Organic Acid Test or OAT is one of my favourite functional tests because of the wealth of information it provides.

Rather like a car mechanic may look at exhaust emissions testing to assess how well an engine is working, so the OAT enables you to have a snapshot of the efficiency of your own metabolic processes.

All that is required is a urine sample taken first thing in the morning. Analysis of the metabolites contained within highlight any potential imbalances and suggestions will be made regarding additional nutritional support tailored to you. This tests covers:

Cellular energy production: the test looks in detail at the steps within cellular energy production, or the Krebs cycle, which was discussed in Chapter Seven. It helps to pinpoint any potential blockages within energy production and thus can be specific about useful nutritional intervention.

Functional B vitamin sufficiency: in particular markers for B12 and folate, both of which are critical nutrients for a process called methylation. Sub-optimal methylation can contribute to raised levels of an amino acid homocysteine, in itself a risk factor for cancer.[193]

Neurotransmitter, or brain chemical, metabolites: including those of adrenalin (stress hormone), dopamine (reward & motivation) and serotonin (happy hormone). On occasion this has helped to highlight a need for additional self care or support, even when the person appears on the outside to be managing well emotionally.

Oxidative damage and antioxidant markers: two metabolites, including 8-Hydroxy-2-deoxyguanosine which was mentioned in Chapter

One, indicate whether your current antioxidant needs are being met.

Phase 1 and phase 2 detoxification capacity: this gives an indication of whether you might benefit from additional detoxification support.

Bowel health: pathogenic bacteria and yeasts produce metabolites which, if present, can be detected in the urine. Although not as detailed as a Gastro Intestinal stool test, this does indicate the extent to which a digestive health programme would be beneficial.

Cost: £220 - £320 (urine)

SpectraCell

An alternative way to assess for nutritional insufficiencies is via the blood. SpectraCell measure the function of 35 nutritional components including vitamins, minerals, antioxidants and amino acids within the white blood cells.

An easy to read report gives information about individual nutrient insufficiencies and enables your practitioner to design a targeted supplement repletion programme.

Cost: c £440 (blood)

Gastro Intestinal Testing

The stool test is the most efficient way to determine the microbial composition of your digestive system. The tests available privately offer far more information than is currently available on the NHS, and is particularly useful if you have a history of digestive issues. This enables you to be specific in respect of a recovery programme.

Typically there are a number of tests available, all of which utilise a number of stool samples. The most basic is a comprehensive parasitology and this yields information about the levels of bacteria (both good and pathogenic), yeasts and parasites present.

Your practitioner can then advise which supplements are most effective against the presenting organisms, and also how to build up the levels of good bacteria through probiotics and fermented foods.

The main lab that I use is Genova, and their standard profile doesn't test for Helicobactor Pylori. If such an infection is suspected (history of ulcers, long term ant-acid use, stomach pain, stomach cancer) then this is available as an add on via stool or breath test. The benefit of the stool test is that proton pump inhibitor (PPI) medication can be continued, whereas the breath test requires that they be stopped for two weeks prior to testing. It is also possible to request H Pylori testing via your GP.

More advanced testing includes an additional number of markers for digestive health. These include information on your digestive capacity and how well you are breaking down fats and fibres, and whether you are producing sufficient digestive enzymes. It can advise whether there is inflammation in the gut (mucus, lactoferrin, calprotectin, eosinophil protein X) or blood, which could be indicative of a more serious condition (in which case I would refer you to your GP).

Testing can also analyse metabolic activity in the gut to ensure that there are sufficient short chain fatty acids. These are produced by the good bacteria and are an energy source for digestive cells. A very useful marker is beta glucuronidase, an enzyme released from certain pathogenic bacteria. It has been implicated in the increased recirculation of toxins, steroid hormones, drugs and carcinogens. This enzyme has the potential to deconjugate potential toxins, preventing their excretion from the body (ie: it interferes with the detoxification process). Studies suggest a link with beta-glucuronidase and cancer.[194] Finally, it can assess for a number of bile acids in the stool. Excessive levels may be associated with risk of gallstones and cancer.

Cost: £150 - £280 (stool)

Functional Immunology and Autoimmunity (Cyrex)

Cyrex labs are world leaders in blood tests which detect an immune reaction to foods, in particular gluten, autoimmune activity in the body and an advanced test for intestinal permeability (leaky gut).

Coeliac disease is an autoimmune disorder of the small intestine caused by gluten and occurs in genetically predisposed people. It is potentially a serious condition because the gut wall becomes damaged and inflamed, and nutrient absorption can be affected. Furthermore the production of antibodies (an immune reaction) can lead to wider auto-immune activity, which is when the body tissues are attacked by the immune system. Health conditions also associated with coeliac include type 1 diabetes, ulcerative colitis and neurological disorders such as epilepsy.

Standard protocol uses blood tests to identify people who may have coeliac disease followed by a biopsy to confirm diagnosis. It generally tests for antibodies against gliadin, a protein within wheat, and Tissue Transglutaminase 2 (tTG2). These are a family of enzymes involving protein polymers, rather like scaffolding, which form barriers and stable structures in tissues. Activation of antibodies to tTGs confirms an auto-immune response.

It is very common for people presenting with symptoms of gluten sensitivity, which resolve when they eliminate wheat, to test negative for coeliac disease.

Enter Cyrex. Their wheat/gluten reactivity and autoimmunity profile assesses for twenty-four antibodies against twelve different wheat fractions and tTGs. Hence it is considerably more sensitive than standard testing and can identify both those with autoimmune activity (coeliac) and those with non-coeliac gluten sensitivity.

Given that coeliac disease presents in people of all ages (my own father was diagnosed at 72 after a lifetime of digestive distress) it is feasible that an earlier elimination of gluten in sensitive people could be very helpful.

Cyrex also offer related tests, including detection of the presence of antibodies to cross reactive foods (including milk, eggs, spelt and other grains) and those confirming autoimmune activity against specific organ tissue. These can appear up to 10 years before the clinical onset of disease, and hence enables early intervention by restricting the consumption of offending foods.

If you are at all concerned about gluten sensitivity or you have significant digestive issues, I encourage you to consider investing in Cyrex testing. Unfortunately you do need to be eating wheat for 14 days prior to testing, which makes it difficult if you have already eliminated gluten.

Cost: £400- £1000

Hormone Testing

This test assesses your metabolism of oestrogens and is recommended for women concerned about hormonal symptoms including menopause and breast cancer risk.

It is a urine test. The more basic version assesses for levels of the five oestrogen metabolites which were discussed in Chapter Seven. These show whether you are accumulating the less desirable forms and pinpoints nutritional support which can improve your ratio of favourable metabolites.

The comprehensive test also includes assessments of levels of the three oestrogens.

Hormone testing can be used alongside Tamoxifen, Herceptin and HRT. However it is not recommended with aromatase inhibitors as these prevent oestrogen production.

Cost: £114 - £254

Essential Fatty Acids (EFAs)

EFAs are critical for cell membrane structure and function and local hormonal signalling. They are transformed into hormone like messengers called prostaglandins, which regulate all stages of inflammation and play a role in enabling the immune system to repair and protect itself.

Unfortunately the dietary intake of EFAs can be severely compromised. Natural sources of omega 3, for instance in meat, is reduced by the regular use of omega 6 grains in animal feeds. There is also a high prevalence of omega 6 oils in the human food supply, from margarines to the ubiquitous vegetable oils which are so widely used in the food industry.

This test evaluates the level of red cell membrane fatty acids, imbalances of which significantly affect inflammatory and other disorders. By knowing the various fatty acid levels, one can re-establish a balance using nutritional supplements.

£180 - £200 (blood)

Adrenal Stress Index (ASI)

The ASI is a good test for someone with a busy and/or stressful lifestyle and is concerned that this might be impacting on their health, or someone who is experiencing very low energy levels, low immunity or continual infections.

It takes a measurement of salivary cortisol at 4 times throughout the day – first thing in the morning, noon, mid-afternoon and before bed. It also measures DHEA, which is another steroid hormone that can become depleted if cortisol levels are significantly elevated over a long period of time. Abnormal DHEA levels are an early indicator of adrenal irregularity.

Cortisol levels are governed by the sleep-wake cycle and should peak early in the morning. A normal output would see a gradual fall in cortisol throughout the day with lowest levels before bed.

Elevated levels at one or more points in the day may indicate the start of adrenal dysfunction and lifestyle remedies play a key role in reducing stress, along with supplements to replace the nutrients which may become depleted with high stress output. If the stressors continue unabated, then DHEA levels may become affected, potentially progressing to one or more cortisol readings recording below range.

Adrenal fatigue is a condition where cortisol levels are consistently below normal levels and this is accompanied by a general sense of being unwell, tired and feeling that you need stimulants such as coffee to prop you up during the day.

So, if high stress is suspected, the ASI can give information on whereabouts you are on the pathway to adrenal issues, and appropriate support can then be discussed.

Cost: £80- £125

Working with a Practitioner

The idea behind this book is to empower and encourage you to create your best health ever, even if you are currently going through a serious health challenge, like cancer. I truly believe that the better our bodies are nourished, the better they can function and that helps whether you are focussing on prevention or recovery.

Much of the information contained within this book can be applied directly. However, there can also be a real benefit in working with a practitioner to help establish the best nutritional plan and supplement regime for you:

1. You have an interested partner who can discuss, debate and guide you. There is a lot of information out there, some of it conflicting. You need to be able to sort out the wheat from the chaff, and explore opinions without feeling bogged down or stressed.

2. They have a wider perspective, working with many people over the course of a week or a year. This helps to bridge the gap between pure theory and practice, as they are continually learning from what works and what doesn't.

3. Their experience can help to home in on your priorities, so that you get the best results without missing important avenues or wasting time and money on things that are less relevant.

4. Your practitioner should be able to check compatibility of recommended supplements with your medications, and liaise with your oncologist or doctor as required.

5. They can recommend and order lab tests on your behalf, interpret the results and make appropriate recommendations.

6. Regular appointments, whether in person or via phone / skype, provide valuable interludes to reflect on your health programme, how it's working and what adjustments should be made.

Finding a Nutritional Practitioner

In the UK one of the main sources of leads for Nutritionists is via the British Association for Applied Nutrition & Nutritional Therapy (www.BANT.org.uk).

In the future, we plan to offer listings of practitioners who have undertaken specific training in working with cancer patients via the website www.InspiredNutrition.co.uk.

The best source of integrative Doctors or clinics is via the directory on the Yes to Life website (www.yestolife.org.uk)

Personal recommendation and word of mouth is another good way to find a reputable practitioner.

How I Work

I work with people nutritionally across a range of health conditions, whether that has currently manifested as a disease condition like cancer, or is merely a cluster of symptoms without a diagnosis. Nutrition is so effective preventatively that working at an early stage can have significant benefits in improving overall wellbeing and can also massively reduce disease risk.

Nutritional therapy is an adjunct to medical care, and so it is important that it works alongside your medical treatment. At a first consultation, which can be in person or over skype / phone, we discuss your health goals and review your health history. With my health detective hat on I will be looking to tease out imbalances which may be contributing to your symptoms.

I ask about your attitude to making changes, whether you are interested in taking supplements, adjusting your lifestyle or investing in additional tests. From here I aim to explain how nutrition may be impacting on your symptoms and we agree a plan for working together.

I also offer workshops under the *Outsmart Cancer* name where you can learn more about cancer and how to make life difficult for it in a safe, motivating and upbeat environment. These are open to both cancer patients and those interested in prevention. The workshops have been generously supported by the charity Together Against Cancer, www.togetheragainstcancer.org.uk.

Together with my colleague Jeraldine Curran, we also offer the *Outsmart Cancer* cookery workshop and are working with Yes to Life, www.yestolife.org.uk to deliver a programme of events this year. We are very grateful for the funding and support that Yes to Life provide.

You can find out more about working privately with me, or attending the workshops that we run at Inspired Nutrition. You may also like to keep updated with nutrition and health information by subscribing to our newsletter from the home page.

Summary

This chapter encourages you to consider a more in depth way of working either in prevention or recovery to individualise your nutritional programme by working with a practitioner. You now have an overview of the kind of testing available privately to supplement your current medical care, should you wish to.

Whilst we are privileged to have a very solid health service available to all, our health is so paramount to our own wellbeing and longevity that it only makes good sense to invest additionally, should you choose to do so. Even just buying this book is of immense benefit if it enables you to tread a more healthful path.

We are working to provide group workshops and cookery classes so that more people have access to local support, and are very grateful to the charities Yes to Life and Together Against Cancer for providing funding to help make this a reality. In the future, we hope that this can be offered more extensively, and are in a position to scale up by training more practitioners to work with us.

I wish you every success in achieving good health and happiness.

Resources

Finding a Qualified Nutritionist

www.BANT.org.uk

www.InspiredNutrition.co.uk

Cancer Support

www.OutsmartCancer.co.uk

www.YesToLife.org.uk

www.TogetherAgainstCancer.org.uk

www.pennybrohncancercare.org

www.canceractive.com

Healthy Food Companies

Grain free, dairy free mixes for breads and cake –
www.UGGfoods.co.uk

Fermented foods – www.CulturedProbiotics.co.uk

Raw milk – www.hookandson.co.uk

Fresh cold pressed linseed oil - www.thelinseedfarm.co.uk

Organic Produce

Information about pesticide residues - www.ewg.org.uk

Riverford Organic Farms - www.riverford.co.uk

Abel and Cole - www.abelandcole.co.uk

Kitchen Gadgets

Juicers, spiralizers, dehydrators and more - www.UKJuicers.com

Fermentation starter kits - www.happykombucha.co.uk

Nut milk bag – www.amazon.co.uk

Kitchen tools – www.pamperedchef.co.uk

Detox Supplies

Enema kits – www.manifesthealth.co.uk

Rebounders and dry skin brush – www.amazon.co.uk

Mindfulness

Online meditations – www.InMindInBody.com

Laughter yoga – www.robertrivest.com

Natural Skincare Ranges

Defiant Beauty - www.jenniferyoung.co.uk

Neal's Yard Remedies - www.nealsyardremedies.com

Useful Websites

www.InspiredNutrition.co.uk

www.chrisbeatcancer.com

www.foodmatters.tv

Recommended Reading

Radical Remission: Surviving Cancer Against All Odds
by Kelly Turner PhD

The Rainbow Diet by Chris Woollams

Vital Signs for Cancer by Dr Xandria Williams

Anticancer: A New Way of Life by David Servan-Schreiber

Personal Stories

What we did to Beat Cancer by Robert Olifent

Mum's Not Having Chemo by Laura Bond

The Adventures of a Cancer Maverick by Nina Joy

A Time to Heal by Beata Bishop

Cookery Books

Against All Grain: Gluten Free, Grain Free & Dairy Free Recipes for Daily Life by Danielle Walker

Honestly Healthy: Eat With Your Body in Mind, the Alkaline Way by Natasha Corrett & Vicki Edgson

The Nourished Kitchen: Farm-to-Table Recipes for the Traditional Foods Lifestyle by Jennifer McGruther

Nourish: Penny Brohn Cancer Care with Christine Bailey

Zest for Life: The Meditteranean Anti-Cancer Diet by Conner Middelmann-Whitney

Healing Foods, Healthy Foods by Gloria Halim

Worth Watching

TED Talk - *Minding your Mitochondria* Dr Terry Wahls

TED Talk - *Can We Eat to Starve Cancer?* by Dr William Li

TED Talk - *The Best Gift I Ever Survived* by Stacey Kramer

TED Talk - *Mind Over Medicine*: Scientific Proof You Can Heal Yourself by Dr Lissa Rankin

You Tube - *Augmenting Cancer Therapy with Diet* by Dr Colin E Champ

You Tube - *Cancer From a Physicist's Perspective, a New Theory of Cancer* by Paul Davies

References

[1] Kelly A. Turner. (2014) Radical Remission, surviving cancer against all odds. Harper One.

[2] Plant J.(Revised 2007) Your Life in Your Hands. Virgin books

[3] Olivier S (2000) The Breast Cancer Prevention & Recovery Diet. Penguin

[4] Davies P Cancer from a physicist's perspective: a new theory of cancer www.youtube.com New Scientist (accessed 26.10.14).

[5] Preetha Anand, Ajaikumar B. Kunnumakara, Chitra Sundaram, Kuzhuvelil B. Harikumar, Sheeja T. Tharakan, Oiki S. Lai, Bokyung Sung, and Bharat B. Aggarwa. (2008) Cancer is a Preventable Disease that Requires Major Lifestyle Changes Pharm Res. Sep; 25(9): 2097–2116

[6] Ahmad AS, Ormiston-Smith N, Sasieni PD (2015)Trends in the lifetime risk of developing cancer in Great Britain: comparison of risk for those born from 1930 to 1960. British Journal of Cancer advance online publication 3 February 2015;

[7] www.macmillan.org.uk Key Statistics Accessed 21/2/15

[8] www.cancerresearchuk.org All cancers combined Key Stats Accessed 21/2/15

[9] https://www.gov.uk/government/policies/helping-more-people-survive-cancer Accessed 21/2/15

[10] http://www.cancer.gov/cancertopics/factsheet/NCI/research-funding Accessed 22/2/15

[11] Preetha Anand, Ajaikumar B. Kunnumakara, Chitra Sundaram, Kuzhuvelil B. Harikumar, Sheeja T. Tharakan, Oiki S. Lai, Bokyung Sung, and Bharat B. Aggarwa. (2008) Cancer is a Preventable Disease that Requires Major Lifestyle Changes Pharm Res. Sep; 25(9): 2097–2116

[12] Cuzick J, Forbes J, Edwards R, Baum M, Cawthorn S, Coates A, Hamed A, Howell A, Powles T; IBIS investigators. (2002) First results from the International Breast Cancer Intervention Study (IBIS-I): a randomised prevention trial. Lancet.Sep 14;360(9336):817-24.

[13] World Cancer Research Fund (2007) Food, Nutrition, Physical Activity and Cancer – A Global Perspective. The American Institute for Cancer Research.

[14] Hanahan D, Weinberg RA (2011) Hallmarks of Cancer: The Next Generation. Cell 144, March 4

[15] World Cancer Research Fund (2007) Food, Nutrition, Physical Activity and Cancer – A Global Perspective. The American Institute for Cancer Research

[16] Wu LL, Chiou CC, Chang PY, Wu JT. (2004) Urinary 8-OHdG: a marker of oxidative stress to DNA and a risk factor for cancer, atherosclerosis and diabetics. Clin Chim Acta. Jan;339(1-2):1-9

[17] He H, Zhao Y, Wang N, Zhang L, Wang C. (2014) 8-Hydroxy-2'-deoxyguanosine expression predicts outcome of esophageal cancer. Ann Diagn Pathol

[18] Coussens LM, Werb Z. (2002) Inflammation and cancer. Nature. Dec 19-26;420(6917):860-7

[19] Allin KH, Nordestgaard BG, Flyger H, Bojesen SE. (2011) Elevated pre-treatment levels of plasma C-reactive protein are associated with poor prognosis after breast cancer: a cohort study. Breast Cancer Res. Jun 3;13(3):R55

[20] Patel C, Ghanim H, Ravishankar S, Sia CL, Viswanathan P, Mohanty P, Dandona P. (2007) Prolonged reactive oxygen species generation and nuclear factor-kappaB activation after a high-fat, high-carbohydrate meal in the obese. J Clin Endocrinol Metab. Nov;92(11):4476-9

[21] Dickinson S, Hancock DP, Petocz P, Ceriello A, Brand-Miller J. (2008) High-glycemic index carbohydrate increases nuclear factor-kappaB activation in mononuclear cells of young, lean healthy subjects. Am J Clin Nutr. May;87(5):1188-93

[22] Li Y, Zhang T. (2014) Targeting cancer stem cells by curcumin and clinical applications. Cancer Lett. May 1;346(2):197-205

[23] Key T, Appleby P, Barnes I, Reeves G. (2002) Endogenous sex hormones and breast cancer in postmenopausal women: reanalysis of nine prospective studies. J Natl Cancer Inst. Apr 17;94(8):606-16.

[24] Key TJ et al. (2013) Sex hormones and risk of breast cancer in premenopausal women: a collaborative reanalysis of individual participant data from seven prospective studies. Lancet Oncol. Sep;14(10):1009-19

[25] Key TJ et al. (2011) Circulating sex hormones and breast cancer risk factors in postmenopausal women: reanalysis of 13 studies. Br J Cancer. Aug 23;105(5):709-22

[26] Wroblewski LE, Peek RM Jr, Wilson KT. (2010) Helicobacter pylori and gastric cancer: factors that modulate disease risk. Clin Microbiol Rev. Oct;23(4):713-39

[27] Hanson KM1, Gratton E, Bardeen CJ. (2006) Sunscreen enhancement of UV-induced reactive oxygen species in the skin. Free Radic Biol Med. Oct 15;41(8):1205-12

[28] National Cancer Institute www.cancer.gov/cancertopics/factsheet/Risk/acrylamide-in-food#r11 (accessed 26.10.14).

[29] Xu Y1, Cui B2, Ran R3, Liu Y3, Chen H4, Kai G5, Shi J6. (2014) Risk assessment, formation, and mitigation of dietary acrylamide: current status and future prospects. Food Chem Toxicol. Jul;69:1-12

[30] www.royalmarsden.nhs.uk Eating Well When You Have Cancer Accessed 19/2/15

[31] The NHS Cancer Plan (2000)

[32] WCRF (2007) Food, Nutrition, Physical Activity and the Prevention of Cancer. American Institute for Cancer Research

[33] Anand P1, Kunnumakkara AB, Sundaram C, Harikumar KB, Tharakan ST, Lai OS, Sung B, Aggarwal BB. (2008) Cancer is a preventable disease that requires major lifestyle changes. Pharm Res. 2008 Sep;25(9):2097-116.

[34] Ornish D et al,(2005) Journal of Urology Sep; 174(3):1065-9

[35] www.KrisCarr.com Accessed 19/2/15

[36] www.ChrisBeatCancer.com Accessed 19/2/15

[37] Turner K (2014) Radical Remission: surviving cancer against all odds. Harper One

[38] Glade MJ. Food, nutrition, and the prevention of cancer: a global perspective. American institute for cancer research/world cancer research fund, American Institute for Cancer Research, 1997. Nutrition. 1999;15:523–526

[39] Pelucchi C, Bosetti C, Rossi M, Negri E, La Vecchia C. (2009) Selected aspects of Mediterranean diet and cancer risk. Nutr Cancer.;61(6):756-66.

[40] Whalen KA, McCullough M, Flanders WD, Hartman TJ, Judd S, Bostick RM. (2014) Paleolithic and Mediterranean diet pattern scores and risk of incident, sporadic colorectal adenomas. Am J Epidemiol. Dec 1;180(11):1088-97.

[41] Le LT, Sabaté J (2014) Beyond meatless, the health effects of vegan diets: findings from the Adventist cohorts.Nutrients.May 27;6(6):2131-47.

[42] Myles IA (2014) Fast food fever: reviewing the impacts of the Western diet on immunity. Nutr J.Jun 17;13:61.

[43] http://www.drugs.com/pro/lansoprazole.html Accessed 9/4/15

[44] Dreizen S1, McCredie KB, Keating MJ, Andersson BS (1990) Nutritional deficiencies in patients receiving cancer chemotherapy. Postgrad Med. 1990 Jan;87(1):163-7, 170.

[45] Block KI, Koch AC, Mea MN, Tothy PK, Newman RA, Gyllenhaal C (2008) Impact of antioxidant supplementation on chemotherapeutic toxicity: A systematic review of the evidence from randomized controlled trials Int. J. Cancer: 123, 1227–1239

[46] Simone CB 2nd1, Simone NL, Simone V, Simone CB. (2007) Antioxidants and other nutrients do not interfere with chemotherapy or radiation therapy and can increase kill and increase survival, part 1. Altern Ther Health Med. Jan-Feb;13(1):22-8.

[47] http://www.nytimes.com/2015/02/21/opinion/when-the-government-tells-you-what-to-eat.html?_r=0

[48] Herbert F Helander, and Lars Fändriks. (2014) Surface area of the digestive tract – revisited Gastrointestinal anatomy. June; 49(6): 681-689

[49] Furness JB, Kunze WA, Clerc N. (1999) Nutrient tasting and signaling mechanisms in the gut. II. The intestine as a sensory organ: neural, endocrine, and immune responses. Am J Physiol. Nov;277(5 Pt 1):G922-8

[50] Peng L1, Li ZR, Green RS, Holzman IR, Lin J. (2009) Butyrate enhances the intestinal barrier by facilitating tight junction assembly via activation of AMP-activated protein kinase in Caco-2 cell monolayers. J Nutr. Sep;139(9):1619-25

[51] Kan Shida and Koji Nomoto (2013). Probiotics as efficient immunopotentiators: Translational role in cancer prevention. Indian J Med Res. November; 138(5): 808–814.

[52] Riina A Kekkonen, Netta Lummela, Heli Karjalainen, Sinikka Latvala, Soile Tynkkynen, Salme Järvenpää, Hannu Kautiainen, Ilkka Julkunen, Heikki Vapaatalo, and Riitta Korpela (2008) Probiotic intervention has strain-specific anti-inflammatory effects in healthy adults. World J Gastroenterol. Apr 7; 14(13): 2029–2036

[53] P Österlund, T Ruotsalainen, R Korpela, M Saxelin, A Ollus, P Valta, M Kouri, I Elomaa, and H Joensuu (2007) Lactobacillus supplementation for diarrhoea related to chemotherapy of colorectal cancer: a randomised study. Br J Cancer. Oct 22; 97(8): 1028–1034.

[54] P Delia, G Sansotta and G Famularo (2007) Use of probiotics for prevention of radiation-induced diarrhea World Journal of Gastroenterology February 14; 13(6): 912–915

[55] World Cancer Research Fund 2012

[56] Chambial S, Dwivedi S, Shukla KK, John PJ, Sharma P. (2013) Vitamin C in disease prevention and cure: an overview. Indian J Clin Biochem. Oct;28(4):314-28

[57] Cameron E, Pauling L. (1976) Supplemental ascorbate in the supportive treatment of cancer: Prolongation of survival times in terminal human cancer. Proc Natl Acad Sci Oct;73(10):3685-9

[58] Kim JE1, Cho HS, Yang HS, Jung DJ, Hong SW, Hung CF, Lee WJ, Kim D. (2012) Depletion of ascorbic acid impairs NK cell activity against ovarian cancer in a mouse model. Immunobiology. 2012 Sep;217(9):873-81

[59] http://www.cancer.gov/cancertopics/pdq/cam/highdosevitaminc/patient/page2 accessed 2/11/14

[60] Ma Y, Chapman J, Levine M, Polireddy K, Drisko J, Chen Q. (2014) High-dose parenteral ascorbate enhanced chemosensitivity of ovarian cancer and reduced toxicity of chemotherapy. Sci Transl Med. Feb 5;6(222).

[61] Close GL, Leckey J, Patterson M, Bradley W, Owens DJ, Fraser WD, Morton JP (2013) The effects of vitamin D(3) supplementation on serum total 25[OH]D concentration and physical performance: a randomised dose-response study. Br J Sports Med. Jul;47(11):692-6

[62] P. J. Goodwin, M. Ennis, K. I. Pritchard, J. Koo and N. Hood (2008) Frequency of vitamin D deficiency at breast cancer diagnosis and association with risk of distant recurrence and death in a prospective cohort study of T1–3, N0–1, M0 B Journal of Clinical Oncology, ASCO Annual Meeting Proceedings (Post-Meeting Edition). Vol 26, No 15S (May 20 Supplement): 511

[63] Assa A1, Vong L2, Pinnell LJ2, Avitzur N2, Johnson-Henry KC2, Sherman PM3. (2014)nVitamin D deficiency promotes epithelial barrier dysfunction and intestinal inflammation. J Infect Dis. 2014 Oct 15;210(8):1296-305.

[64] Khalsa S (2009) The Vitamin D Revolution Hay House

[65] Powell M. (2013) Medicinal Mushrooms – the essential guide. Bamboo publishing.

[66] Jeong SC, Koyyalamudi SR, Jeong YT, Song CH, Pang G. (2012) Macrophage immunomodulating and antitumor activities of polysaccharides isolated from Agaricus bisporus white button mushrooms. J Med Food. 2012 Jan;15(1):58-65

[67] Kidd PM. (2000) The use of mushroom glucans and proteoglycans in cancer treatment. Altern Med Rev. Feb;5(1):4-27

[68] Jiang J1, Slivova V, Valachovicova T, Harvey K, Sliva D. (2004) Ganoderma lucidum inhibits proliferation and induces apoptosis in human prostate cancer cells PC-3. Int J Oncol. May;24(5):1093-9

[69] Bojana Boh, Marin Berovic, Jingsong Zhang, Lin Zhi-Bin. (2007) *Ganoderma lucidum* and its pharmaceutically active compounds. Biotechnology Annual Review. 13(1):265–301

[70] Alejandro Cuevas, Nicolás Saavedra, Luis A. Salazar, and Dulcineia S. P. Abdalla. (2013) Modulation of Immune Function by Polyphenols: Possible Contribution of Epigenetic Factors. Nutrients. Jul; 5(7): 2314–2332

[71] Mineva ND, Paulson KE, Naber SP, Yee AS, Sonenshein GE (2013) Epigallocatechin-3-gallate inhibits stem-like inflammatory breast cancer cells. PLoS One. Sep 11;8(9)

[72] Golombick T, Diamond TH, Manoharan A, Ramakrishna R. (2012) Monoclonal gammopathy of undetermined significance, smoldering multiple myeloma, and curcumin: a randomized, double-blind placebo-controlled cross-over 4g study and an open-label 8g extension study. Am J Hematol. May;87(5):455-60

[73] Belcaro G, Hosoi M, Pellegrini L, Appendino G, Ippolito E, Ricci A, Ledda A, Dugall M, Cesarone MR, Maione C, Ciammaichella G, Genovesi D, Togni S. (2014) A controlled study of a lecithinized delivery system of curcumin (Meriva®) to alleviate the adverse effects of cancer treatment. Phytother Res. Mar;28(3):444-50

[74] Paller CJ, Ye X, Wozniak PJ, Gillespie BK, Sieber PR, Greengold RH, Stockton BR, Hertzman BL, Efros MD, Roper RP, Liker HR, Carducci MA. (2013) A randomized phase II study of pomegranate extract for men with rising PSA following initial therapy for localized prostate cancer. Prostate Cancer Prostatic Dis. Mar;16(1):50-5

[75] Thomas R (2009) Your Lifestyle After Cancer. Health Education Publications

[76] Thomas R, Williams M, Sharma H, Chaudry A, Bellamy P. (2014) A double-blind, placebo-controlled randomised trial evaluating the effect of a polyphenol-rich whole food supplement on PSA progression in men with prostate cancer--the U.K. NCRN Pomi-T study. Prostate Cancer Prostatic Dis. Jun;17(2):180-6

[77] Martínez-Zaguilán R, Seftor EA, Seftor RE, Chu YW, Gillies RJ, Hendrix MJ. (1996) Acidic pH enhances the invasive behavior of human melanoma cells. Clin Exp Metastasis. Mar;14(2):176-86.

[78] Moellering RE, Black KC, Krishnamurty C, Baggett BK, Stafford P, Rain M, Gatenby RA, Gillies RJ. (2008) Acid treatment of melanoma cells selects for invasive phenotypes. Clin Exp Metastasis. 2008;25(4):411-25.

[79] https://www.gdx.net/uk/patients Accessed 23/2/15

[80] Aihara H ((1986) Acid & Alkaline. George Ohsawa Macrobiotic Foundation

[81] Lustig R www.youtube.com Sugar: The Bitter Truth (accessed 12/2/15)

[82] Daily Mail 'How much hidden sugar is your diet' 25/2/14

[83] Walker Samuel et al. (2013) In vivo imaging of glucose uptake and metabolism in tumors. Nature Medicine. 19:1067–1072

[84] Masur K, Vetter C, Hinz A, Tomas N, Henrich H, Niggemann B, Zänker KS. (2011) Diabetogenic glucose and insulin concentrations modulate transcriptome and protein levels involved in tumour cell migration, adhesion and proliferation. Br J Cancer. Jan 18;104(2):345-52

[85] Ho VW , Leung K, Hsu A, Luk B, Lai J, Shen SY, Minchinton AI, Waterhouse D, Bally MB, Lin W, Nelson BH, Sly LM, Krystal G. (2011) A low carbohydrate, high protein diet slows tumor growth and prevents cancer initiation. Cancer Res. Jul 1;71(13):4484-93

[86] Lajous M, Boutron-Ruault MC, Fabre A, Clavel-Chapelon F, Romieu I. (2008) Carbohydrate intake, glycemic index, glycemic load, and risk of postmenopausal breast cancer in a prospective study of French women. Am J Clin Nutr. May;87(5):1384-91

[87] Sieri S1, Pala V, Brighenti F, Agnoli C, Grioni S, Berrino F, Scazzina F, Palli D, Masala G, Vineis P, Sacerdote C, Tumino R, Giurdanella MC, Mattiello A, Panico S, Krogh V. (2013) High glycemic diet and breast cancer occurrence in the Italian EPIC cohort. Nutr Metab Cardiovasc Dis. Jul;23(7):628-34

[88] Xandria Williams (2010) Vital Signs for Cancer. Piatkus

[89] Weatherby D & Ferguson S (2002) Blood Chenistry and CBC Analysis. Bear Mountain Publishing

[90]

http://www.macmillan.org.uk/Documents/AboutUs/Commissioners/Movemorereport.pdf Accessed 16/2/15

[91] Xin F, Jiang L, Liu X, Geng C, Wang W, Zhong L, Yang G, Chen M. (2014) Bisphenol A induces oxidative stress-associated DNA damage in INS-1 cells. Mutat Res Genet Toxicol Environ Mutagen. Jul 15;769:29-33

[92] Crinnion WJ. (2011) Sauna as a valuable clinical tool for cardiovascular, autoimmune, toxicant- induced and other chronic health problems. Altern Med Rev. Sep;16(3):215-25

[93] Humphrey LL, Fu R, Buckley DI, Freeman M, Helfand M. (2008) Periodontal disease and coronary heart disease incidence: a systematic review and meta-analysis. J Gen Intern Med. Dec;23(12):2079-86

[94] Rajesh KS, Thomas D, Hegde S, Kumar MS. (2013) Poor periodontal health: A cancer risk? J Indian Soc Periodontol. Nov;17(6):706-10

[95] Hwang IM, Sun LM, Lin CL, Lee CF, Kao CH. (2014) Periodontal disease with treatment reduces subsequent cancer risks. QJM. Oct;107(10):805-12

[96] Kim ES, Chun HJ, Keum B, Seo YS, Jeen YT, Lee HS, Um SH, Kim CD, Ryu HS. (2014) Coffee enema for preparation for small bowel video capsule endoscopy: a pilot study. Clin Nutr Res. Jul;3(2):134-41

[97] Teekachunhatean S, Tosri N, Rojanasthien N, Srichairatanakool S, Sangdee C. (2013) Pharmacokinetics of Caffeine following a Single Administration of Coffee Enema versus Oral Coffee Consumption in Healthy Male Subjects. ISRN Pharmacol.2013:147238

[98] Wright CM. (2011) Biographical notes on Ancel Keys and Salim Yusuf: origins and significance of the seven countries study and the INTERHEART study. J Clin Lipidol. Nov-Dec;5(6):434-40

[99] Gary Taubes. (2007) The Diet Delusion. Random House Books. Location 772

[100] Gary Taubes. (2007) The Diet Delusion. Random House Books. Location 5530

[101] Gary Taubes. (2007) The Diet Delusion. Random House Books. Location 7344

[102] Denise Minger 'Death by Food Pyramid: How Shoddy Science, Sketchy Politics & Shady Special Interests Ruined Your Health

[103] Tom Naughton www.youtube.com 'Diet, Health and the Wisdom of Crowds' Accessed 10/11/14.

[104] Udo Erasmus. (1993) 'Fats that heal, fats that kill' Alive Books

[105] TIME magazine 12 June 2014

[106] Ramsden CE, Zamora D, Leelarthaepin B, Majchrzak-Hong SF, Faurot KR, Suchindran CM, Ringel A, Davis JM, Hibbeln JR. (2013) Use of dietary linoleic acid for secondary prevention of coronary heart disease and death: evaluation of recovered data from the Sydney Diet Heart Study and updated meta-analysis. BMJ. Feb 4;346.

[107] Chang CY1, Ke DS, Chen JY. (2009) Essential fatty acids and human brain. Acta Neurol Taiwan. Dec;18(4):231-41

[108] Hottman DA1, Chernick D2, Cheng S1, Wang Z1, Li L3. (2014) HDL and cognition in neurodegenerative disorders. Neurobiol Dis. Aug 13.

[109] www.dailymail.co.uk (2014) Supermarket ready meals contain TEN TEASPOONS- sugar, accessed 17/2/15

[110] Dr R C Atkins (2003) New Diet Revolution. Random House

[111] Ornish D et al Can lifestyle changes reverse coronary heart disease? The Lifestyle Heart Trial. Lancet 1990 Jul 21;336(8708):129-33

[112] Youngman LD, Campbell TC (1992) Inhibition of Aflatoxin B1-induced GGT positive hepatic preneoplastic foci and tumors by low protein diets: evidence that altered GGT+ foci indicate neoplastic potential. Carcinogenesis . Sep; 13(9):1607-13

[113] T. Colin Campbell (2006) The China Study Benbella Books, Dallas

[114] Minger D The China Study: Fact or Fallacy www.rawfoodsos.com Accessed 16/7/14

[115] Fraser GE (1999) Associations between diet and cancer, ischemic heart disease, and all-cause mortality in non-Hispanic white California Seventh-day Adventists. Am J Clin Nutr. Sep;70(3 Suppl):532S-538S.

[116] Dr Terry Wahls Minding My Mitochondria – TED talk www.youtube.com Accessed 10/11/14

[117] Caruso D Mark Hyman MD, Profile www.lef.org/Magazine/2007/8/profile/Page-01 Accessed 23/2/15

[118] www.againstallgrain.com/about-me/ Accessed 23/2/15

[119] www.thepaleomom.com/about-sarah-2 Accessed 23/2/15

[120] http://www.swankmsdiet.org/ Accessed 23/2/15

[121] Farvid MS, Cho E, Chen WY, Eliassen AH, Willett WC. (2014) Dietary protein sources in early adulthood and breast cancer incidence: prospective cohort study. BMJ. Jun 10;348:g3437

[122] WCRF (2007) Food, Nutrition, Physical Activity and the Prevention of Cancer. American Institute for Cancer Research

[123] L Keith (2009) The Vegetarian Myth – food, justice, sustainability.Flashpoint Press

[124] Plant J.(Revised 2007) Your Life in Your Hands. Virgin books.

[125] Kristjánsson G, Venge P, Hällgren R. Mucosal reactivity to cow's milk protein in Coeliac disease. *Clin Exp Immunol*. 2007; 147(3):449-455

[126] Tate PL1, Bibb R, Larcom LL. Milk stimulates growth of prostate cancer cells in culture. Nutr Cancer. 2011 Nov;63(8):1361-6

[127] Farlow DW1, Xu X, Veenstra TD. Comparison of estrone and 17β-estradiol levels in commercial goat and cow milk. J Dairy Sci. 2012 Apr;95(4):1699-708. doi: 10.3168/jds.2011-5072

[128] Attaie R1, Richter RL Size distribution of fat globules in goat milk. J Dairy Sci. 2000 May;83(5):940

[129] www.nhs.co.uk A Balanced Diet Accessed 18 July 2014

[130] Perlmutter D (2014) Grain Brain. Yellow Kite

[131] Davis W (2014) Wheat Belly: lose the wheat, lose the weight and find your path back to health. Harper Collins

[132] de Punder K, Pruimboom L. (2013) The dietary intake of wheat and other cereal grains and their role in inflammation. Nutrients. Mar 12;5(3):771-87

[133] Knott CS, Coombs N, Stamatakis E, Biddulph JP (2015) All cause mortality and the case for age specific alcohol consumption guidelines: pooled analyses of up to 10 population based cohorts. BMJ. Feb 10;350

[134] Seitz HK, Pelucchi C, Bagnardi V, La Vecchia C. (2012) Epidemiology and pathophysiology of alcohol and breast cancer: Update 2012. Alcohol & Alcoholism .May-Jun;47(3):204-12.

[135] Castro GD, Castro JA. (2014) Alcohol drinking and mammary cancer: Pathogenesis and potential dietary preventive alternatives. World J Clin Oncol. 2014 Oct 10;5(4):713-29

[136] Wang Y, Tong J, Chang B, Wang B, Zhang D, Wang B. (2014) Effects of alcohol on intestinal epithelial barrier permeability and expression of tight junction-associated proteins. Mol Med Rep. Jun;9(6):2352-6. doi: 10.3892/mmr.2014.2126. Epub 2014 Apr 9.

[137] http://www.epa.gov/opp00001/pestsales/07pestsales/market_estimates2007.pdf

[138] Barański M, Srednicka-Tober D, Volakakis N, Seal C, Sanderson R, Stewart GB, Benbrook C, Biavati B, Markellou E6, Giotis C, Gromadzka-Ostrowska J, Rembiałkowska E, Skwarło-Sońta K, Tahvonen R, Janovská D, Niggli U12, Nicot P, Leifert C. (2014) Higher antioxidant and lower cadmium concentrations and lower incidence of pesticide residues in organically grown crops: a systematic literature review and meta-analyses. Br J Nutr. Sep 14;112(5):794-811.

[139] http://www.ewg.org/foodnews/index.php Accessed 29/3/15

[140] Mineva ND, Paulson KE, Naber SP, Yee AS, Sonenshein GE. (2013) Epigallocatechin-3-gallate inhibits stem-like inflammatory breast cancer cells. PLoS One.Sep 11;8(9)

[141] http://www.soilassociation.org/Whatisorganic/Organicanimals Accessed 9/4/15

[142] Jing K, Wu T, Lim K. (2013) Omega-3 polyunsaturated fatty acids and cancer. Anticancer Agents Med Chem. Oct;13(8):1162-77

[143] Forsberg ND, Stone D, Harding A, Harper B, Harris S, Matzke MM, Cardenas A, Waters KM, Anderson KA. (2012) Effect of Native American fish smoking methods on dietary exposure to polycyclic aromatic hydrocarbons and possible risks to human health. J Agric Food Chem. Jul 11;60(27):6899-906

[144] https://www.food.gov.uk/business-industry/farmingfood/dairy-guidance/rawmilkcream Accessed 9/4/15

[145] Egner PA et al. (2014) Rapid and sustainable detoxication of airborne pollutants by broccoli sprout beverage: results of a randomized clinical trial in china. Cancer Prev Res (Phila). Aug;7(8):813-23

[146] Woolams C. (2008) The Rainbow Diet. Health Issues Ltd

[147] National Diet & Nutrition Survey (2011)

[148] Rogan EG. (2006) The natural chemopreventive compound indole-3-carbinol: state of the science. In Vivo. Mar-Apr;20(2):221-8

[149] Holzapfel NP, Holzapfel BM, Champ S, Feldthusen J, Clements J, Hutmacher DW. (2013) The potential role of lycopene for the prevention and therapy of prostate cancer: from molecular mechanisms to clinical evidence. Int J Mol Sci. Jul 12;14(7):14620-46

[150] Mason JK. (2010) Flaxseed oil-trastuzumab interaction in breast cancer. Food Chem Toxicol. Aug-Sep;48(8-9):2223-6

[151] Truan JS. (2010) Flaxseed oil reduces the growth of human breast tumors (MCF-7) at high levels of circulating estrogen. Mol Nutr Food Res. Oct;54(10):1414-21

[152] Frenkel M1, Abrams DI, Ladas EJ, Deng G, Hardy M, Capodice JL, Winegardner MF, Gubili JK, Yeung KS, Kussmann H, Block KI

(2013) Integrating dietary supplements into cancer care.

Integr Cancer Ther. Sep;12(5):369-84.

[153] Lindseth GN, Coolahan SE, Petros TV, Lindseth PD. (2014) Neurobehavioral effects of aspartame consumption. Res Nurs Health. Jun;37(3):185-93

[154] Bastard JP, Maachi M, Lagathu C, Kim MJ, Caron M, Vidal H, Capeau J, Feve B. (2006)Recent advances in the relationship between obesity, inflammation, and insulin resistance. Eur Cytokine Netw. Mar;17(1):4-12

[155] Agrawal NK, Kant S. (2014)Targeting inflammation in diabetes: Newer therapeutic options.World J Diabetes. Oct 15;5(5):697-710

[156] Pearson TA, Mensah GA, Alexander RW, Anderson JL, Cannon RO 3rd, Criqui M, Fadl YY, Fortmann SP, Hong Y, Myers GL, Rifai N, Smith SC Jr, Taubert K, Tracy RP, Vinicor F; Centers for Disease Control and Prevention; American Heart Association. (2003) Markers of inflammation and cardiovascular disease: application to clinical and public health practice: A statement for healthcare professionals from the Centers for Disease Control and Prevention and the American Heart Association. Circulation. Jan 28;107(3):499-511

[157] Ghanem FA, Movahed A. (2007) Inflammation in high blood pressure: a clinician perspective. J Am Soc Hypertens. Mar-Apr;1(2):113-9

[158] Hajishengallis G. (2014) Periodontitis: from microbial immune subversion to systemic inflammation. Nat Rev Immunol. Dec 23;15(1):30-44

[159] Berk M, Williams LJ, Jacka FN, O'Neil A, Pasco JA, Moylan S, Allen NB, Stuart AL, Hayley AC, Byrne ML, Maes M. (2013) So depression is an inflammatory disease, but where does the inflammation come from? BMC Med. Sep 12;11:200.

[160] López-Alarcón M, Perichart-Perera O, Flores-Huerta S, Inda-Icaza P, Rodríguez-Cruz M, Armenta-Álvarez A, Bram-Falcón MT, Mayorga-Ochoa M. (2014) Excessive refined carbohydrates and scarce micronutrients intakes increase inflammatory mediators and insulin resistance in prepubertal and pubertal obese children independently of obesity. Mediators Inflamm.:849031

[161] Werawatganon D, Rakananurak N, Sallapant S, Prueksapanich P, Somanawat K, Klaikeaw N, Rerknimitr R. (2014) Aloe vera attenuated gastric injury on indomethacin-induced gastropathy in rats. World J Gastroenterol. Dec 28;20(48):18330-7

[162] Nagpal R, Kaur V, Kumar M, Marotta F. (2012) Effect of Aloe vera juice on growth and activities of Lactobacilli in-vitro. Acta Biomed. Dec;83(3):183-8

[163] Santos AM, Lopes T, Oleastro M, Gato IV, Floch P, Benejat L, Chaves P, Pereira T, Seixas E, Machado J, Guerreiro AS.(2015) Curcumin inhibits gastric inflammation induced by helicobacter pylori infection in a mouse model. Nutrients. Jan 6;7(1):306-20.

[164] Chainani-Wu N. (2003) Safety and anti-inflammatory activity of curcumin: a component of tumeric (Curcuma longa). Altern Complement Med. Feb;9(1):161-8

[165] Simopoulos AP. (2002) Omega-3 fatty acids in inflammation and autoimmune diseases. J Am Coll Nutr. Dec;21(6):495-505

[166] Viswanatha Swamy AH, Patil PA. (2008) Effect of some clinically used proteolytic enzymes on inflammation in rats. Indian J Pharm Sci. Jan;70(1):114-7

[167] Gonzalez NJ, Isaacs L. (2007) The Gonzalez Therapy and Cancer ALTERNATIVE THERAPIES, Jan/Feb; 13(1).

[168] Butel MJ. (2014) Probiotics, gut microbiota and health. Med Mal Infect. Jan;44(1):1-8.

[169] Fasano A, and Shea-Donohue T. (2005) Mechanisms of disease: the role of intestinal barrier function in the pathogenesis of gastrointestinal autoimmune diseases. Nat Clin Pract Gastroenterol Hepatol. Sep;2(9):416-22

[170] Saggioro A. (2014) Leaky gut, microbiota, and cancer: an incoming hypothesis. J Clin Gastroenterol. Nov-Dec;48 Suppl 1:S62-6

[171] Wallock-Richards D, Doherty CJ, Doherty L, Clarke DJ, Place M, and Govan JR, Campopiano DJ. (2014) Garlic Revisited: Antimicrobial Activity of Allicin-Containing Garlic Extracts against Burkholderia cepacia Complex. PLoS One. Dec 1;9(12):e112726

[172] Dabos KJ, Sfika E, Vlatta LJ, Frantzi D, Amygdalos GI, and Giannikopoulos G. (2010)

Is Chios mastic gum effective in the treatment of functional dyspepsia? A prospective randomised double-blind placebo controlled trial. J Ethnopharmacol. Feb 3;127(2):205-9

[173] Miyamoto T, Okimoto T, and Kuwano M. (2014) Chemical Composition of the Essential Oil of Mastic Gum and their Antibacterial Activity Against Drug-Resistant Helicobacter pylori. Nat Prod Bioprospect. Aug;4(4):227-31

[174] APS Hungin, C Mulligan, B Pot, P Whorwell, L Agréus, P Fracasso, C Lionis, J Mendive, J-M Philippart de Foy, G Rubin, C Winchester, and N Wit. (2013) Systematic review: probiotics in the management of lower gastrointestinal symptoms in clinical practice – an evidence-based international guide. Aliment Pharmacol Ther. Oct; 38(8): 864–886

[175] Osterlund P, Ruotsalainen T, Korpela R, Saxelin M, Ollus A, Valta P, Kouri M, Elomaa I, and Joensuu H. (2007) Lactobacillus supplementation for diarrhoea related to chemotherapy of colorectal cancer: a randomised study. Br J Cancer. Oct 22;97(8):1028-34

[176] Lima AA, Anstead GM, Zhang Q, Figueiredo ÍL, Soares AM, Mota RM, Lima NL, Guerrant RL, and Oriá RB. (2014) Effects of glutamine alone or in combination with zinc and vitamin A on growth, intestinal barrier function, stress and satiety-related hormones in Brazilian shantytown children. Clinics (Sao Paulo). Apr; 69(4): 225–233

[177] Kim JW, Jeon WK, Yun JW, Park DI, Cho YK, Sung IK, Sohn CI, Kim BI, Yeom JS, Park HS, Kim EJ, Shin MS. (2005) Protective effects of bovine colostrum on non-steroidal anti-inflammatory drug induced intestinal damage in rats. Asia Pac J Clin Nutr. 2005;14(1):103-7.

[178] Flint MS and Bovbjerg DH. (2012) DNA damage as a result of psychological stress: implications for breast cancer. Breast Cancer Res. Sep 21;14(5):320

[179] Chida Y, Hamer M, Wardle J, and Steptoe A. (2008) Do stress-related psychosocial factors contribute to cancer incidence and survival? Nat Clin Pract Oncol. Aug;5(8):466-75

[180] V.K. Ranganathan, V. Siemionow, J.Z. Lui, V. Sangal, and G.H.Yue. (2004) 'From mental power to muscle power - gaining strength by using the mind'. Neuropyschologia. 42(7): 994-56

[181] Sarah Nechuta, Wei Lu, Zhi Chen, Ying Zheng, Kai Gu, Hui Cai, Wei Zheng, and Xiao Ou Shu. (2011) Vitamin supplement use during breast cancer treatment and survival: a prospective cohort study. Cancer Epidemiol Biomarkers Prev. Feb; 20(2): 262–271

[182] Nicolson GL. (2005) Lipid replacement/antioxidant therapy as an adjunct supplement to reduce the adverse effects of cancer therapy and restore mitochondrial function. Pathol Oncol Res. 11(3):139-44

[183] Richard S. Lord, Bradley Bongiovanni, and J. Alexander Bralley. (2002) Estrogen Metabolism and the Diet-Cancer Connection: Rationale for Assessing the Ratio of Urinary Hydroxylated Estrogen Metabolites. Alternative Medicine Review. May; 7(2):112-29

[184] Lord RS1, Bongiovanni B, Bralley JA. (2002) Estrogen metabolism and the diet-cancer connection: rationale for assessing the ratio of urinary hydroxylated estrogen metabolites. Altern Med Rev. Apr;7(2):112-29.

[185] Sowers MR1, Crawford S, McConnell DS, Randolph JF Jr, Gold EB, Wilkin MK, Lasley B. (2006) Selected diet and lifestyle factors are associated with estrogen metabolites in a multiracial/ethnic population of women.J Nutr. Jun;136(6):1588-95.

[186] Sturgeon SR1, Volpe SL, Puleo E, Bertone-Johnson ER, Heersink J, Sabelawski S, Wahala K, Bigelow C, Kurzer MS. (2010) Effect of flaxseed consumption on urinary levels of estrogen metabolites in postmenopausal women.Nutr Cancer. ;62(2):175-80.

[187] Peters LP1, Teel RW (2003) Effect of high sucrose diet on cytochrome P450 1A and heterocyclic amine mutagenesis. Anticancer Res.Jan-Feb;23(1A):399-403.

[188] Bradlow HL1, Davis DL, Lin G, Sepkovic D, Tiwari R. (1995) Effects of pesticides on the ratio of 16 alpha/2-hydroxyestrone: a biologic marker of breast cancer risk. Environ Health Perspect. 1995 Oct;103 Suppl 7:147-50.

[189] Sung KC1, Ryu S2, Wild SH3, Byrne CD4. (2015) An increased high-density lipoprotein cholesterol/apolipoprotein A-I ratio is associated with increased cardiovascular and all-cause mortality. Heart. 2015 Apr 1;101(7):553-8. doi: 10.1136/heartjnl-2014-306784. Epub 2015 Jan 30.

[190] LAWSON R. (1956) Implications of surface temperatures in the diagnosis of breast cancer.Can Med Assoc J. 1956 Aug 15;75(4):309-11.

[191] Gautherie M, Gros CM. (1980) Breast thermography and cancer risk prediction. Cancer. Jan 1;45(1):51-6.

[192] Williams X (2013) Detecting Cancer. Writersworld, Oxon UK

[193] Keshteli AH1, Baracos VE1, Madsen KL1. (2015) Hyperhomocysteinemia as a potential contributor of colorectal cancer development in inflammatory bowel diseases: A review. World J Gastroenterol.Jan 28;21(4):1081-1090.

[194] Kim DH1, Jin YH (2001) Intestinal bacterial beta-glucuronidase activity of patients with colon cancer. Arch Pharm Res. Dec;24(6):564-7.